Introduction to Health Research Methods

A Practical Guide

Kathryn H. Jacobsen, MPH, PhD
Associate Professor of Epidemiology
George Mason University
Fairfax, Virginia

JONES & BARTLETT
LEARNING

World Headquarters

Jones & Bartlett Learning
40 Tall Pine Drive
Sudbury, MA 01776
978-443-5000
info@jblearning.com
www.jblearning.com

Jones & Bartlett Learning
Canada
6339 Ormindale Way
Mississauga, Ontario L5V 1J2
Canada

Jones & Bartlett Learning
International
Barb House, Barb Mews
London W6 7PA
United Kingdom

Jones & Bartlett Learning books and products are available through most bookstores and online booksellers. To contact Jones & Bartlett Learning directly, call 800-832-0034, fax 978-443-8000, or visit our website, www.jblearning.com.

Substantial discounts on bulk quantities of Jones & Bartlett Learning publications are available to corporations, professional associations, and other qualified organizations. For details and specific discount information, contact the special sales department at Jones & Bartlett Learning via the above contact information or send an email to specialsales@jblearning.com.

This publication is designed to provide accurate and authoritative information in regard to the Subject Matter covered. It is sold with the understanding that the publisher is not engaged in rendering legal, accounting, or other professional service. If legal advice or other expert assistance is required, the service of a competent professional person should be sought.

Production Credits
Publisher: Michael Brown
Editorial Assistant: Teresa Reilly
Associate Production Editor: Kate Stein
Senior Marketing Manager: Sophie Fleck
Manufacturing and Inventory Control Supervisor:
  Amy Bacus

Composition: Achorn International
Art: diacriTech
Cover Design: Kristin E. Parker
Cover Image: © Ivan Mikhaylov/
  Dreamstime.com
Printing and Binding: Malloy, Inc.
Cover Printing: Malloy, Inc.

Library of Congress Cataloging-in-Publication Data
Jacobsen, Kathryn H.
  Introduction to health research methods : a practical guide / Kathryn H. Jacobsen.
    p. ; cm.
  Includes index.
  ISBN-13: 978-0-7637-8334-1 (pbk.)
  ISBN-10: 0-7637-8334-X (pbk.)
  1. Medicine—Research—Methodology. 2. Health—Research—Methodology.
3. Experimental design. I. Title.
  [DNLM: 1. Biomedical Research—methods. 2. Research Design. W 20.5]
  R850.J33 2012
  610.72—dc22

                                                              2011000464

6048
Printed in the United States of America
15 14 13 12 11   10 9 8 7 6 5 4 3 2 1

Contents

CHAPTER 31 ▪ **Writing Strategies**   **239**

CHAPTER 32 ▪ **Critically Revising**   **245**

CHAPTER 33 ▪ **Posters and Presentations**   **249**

CHAPTER 34 ▪ **Selecting Target Journals**   **259**

CHAPTER 35 ▪ The Submission, Review, and Publication Process 263

CHAPTER 36 ▪ Why Publish? 277

Preface

The goal of this book is to make the health research process accessible, manageable, and perhaps even enjoyable for new researchers. One of the reasons that engaging in health research is satisfying is because research is the necessary foundation for meaningful improvements in clinical and public health practice. Research helps us learn how to be healthier and how to help our families, friends, and communities improve and maintain their health.

Without the building blocks provided by health research, there would be no evidence about the risk factors for various disorders, no certainty about whether new vaccines protect against infection, and no ability to identify and map areas that have a high rate of various diseases. There would be no way of knowing which therapies have the best outcomes or whether survival rates for various conditions are improving. And there would be no scientific basis for selecting the tools that most effectively support individual and community health.

But it is not just the outcomes that make research rewarding. The research process itself—the process of exploring the unknown and discovering answers to previously unanswered questions—can be exciting.

This book is a practical, step-by-step guide to the research process.

All research projects follow the same steps: identifying a focused research question, collecting data that will answer the question, analyzing the accumulated evidence, and disseminating the findings. The investigation proceeds through these same basic steps regardless of whether it involves conducting a clinical trial, organizing a neighborhood survey, analyzing an existing dataset, or synthesizing the existing literature through meta-analysis. The same steps are followed whether the researcher is trained in medicine, nursing, public health, physical therapy, psychology, or any other clinical or social science discipline. And the steps are the same regardless of whether the investigator is an undergraduate student or a seasoned professional.

Health research is an intentional process that requires meticulous attention and persistence, but it is not complicated. Anyone who is willing to follow the steps outlined in this guidebook can conceptualize a research project and see it through to completion. And every project, no matter how modest, has the potential to contribute to the knowledge base for the health sciences—and perhaps to eventually translate into improved patient care, enriched organizational effectiveness, and enhanced community health. An increase in the number of active investigators who can conduct conscientious research and accurately communicate their findings to others will benefit us all.

This book is an invitation to make your own contribution to the evidence that will inform future decisions about preventing disease, allocating health resources, and promoting health.

About the Author

Kathryn H. Jacobsen, MPH, PhD, is an associate professor of epidemiology at George Mason University in Fairfax, Virginia. She earned an MPH in International Health and a PhD in Epidemiology from the University of Michigan. Her research portfolio includes field projects in Africa, Asia, and the Americas as well as systematic reviews of the global burden of disease. She has published the results of her research in a variety of journals, including *International Journal of Epidemiology*, *Journal of Health Economics*, *Journal of Medical Ethics*, *Health Promotion International*, and *Vaccine*. She is also the author of *Introduction to Global Health*, published by Jones & Bartlett Learning.

The Purpose and Process of Health Research

Health research is the process of systematically investigating a single well-defined aspect of physical, mental, or social well-being.

■ 1.1 Types of Health Research

Health researchers help in answering many questions. For example:

- Is an 8-week physical therapy program effective at reducing the risk of anterior cruciate ligament tears in high school athletes?
- Is taking a daily multivitamin associated with a decreased risk of colon cancer?
- What are the most common signs and symptoms associated with multiple sclerosis?
- How common is skin cancer among adults living in California?
- Are statins as effective at lowering cholesterol in women as they are in men?
- According to women receiving mammograms, what factors most influenced their decision to seek out routine breast cancer screening?
- Are the annual incidence rates of bacterial meningitis different in Argentina, Kenya, and Thailand?
- How much does the risk of severe hearing loss increase with age?
- Which factors predict binge drinking behavior in college and university students?

- Did the health department's campaign to promote flu shots change the opinions and behavior of county residents?

Research is the process of systematically and carefully investigating a subject in order to learn or discover new information about the world. Most research focuses on a relatively small population. However, the goal of researchers—especially those who publish their findings in an academic or professional journal—is often to identify trends or to develop new theories or methods that are generalizable or that can be more broadly applied.

Health is a construct that extends over all aspects of physical, mental, and social well-being. *Health researchers* examine the biological, socioeconomic, and environmental factors that contribute to health and to disease, illness, disability, and death. *Health research* encompasses studies ranging from laboratory research (e.g., molecular biology, microbiology, immunology, and genetics), to clinical trials (e.g., studies in surgery, pharmacology, and physical therapy), to broad surveys of global health and public health policy. As the word "laboratory" implies, *laboratory studies* are typically conducted in the controlled environment of a special research facility, whereas the data for *population-based studies* are typically conducted using human subjects (FIGURE 1-1).

This book focuses on population-level health research, which encompasses most clinical and public health research (FIGURE 1-2). Population health research objectives may include, along with many others:

- Identifying and classifying new health problems
- Determining risk factors for disease

Examples of Laboratory Research	Examples of Population Research
• Compare tests of air quality in several metropolitan areas	• Compare rates of acute lung diseases in several metropolitan areas and see whether the rates of disease are correlated with local air quality
• Analyze the biochemical composition of selected foods	• Use a food frequency questionnaire to examine dietary behaviors in a selected population group
• Identify biological mechanisms for the emergence of drug-resistant strains of bacteria	• Identify the risk factors for acquiring a drug-resistant bacterial infection
• Identify genes that might be linked to an increased risk of breast cancer	• Determine whether survival following a breast cancer diagnosis is linked to the presence of certain genes
• Develop a new vaccine	• Conduct a vaccine trial

FIGURE 1-1 Comparison of Laboratory and Population Health Research

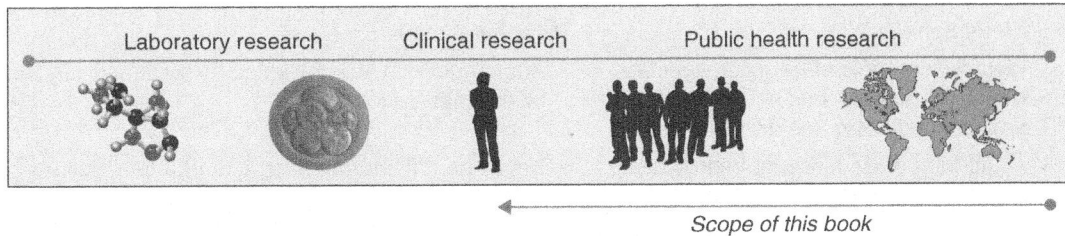

FIGURE 1-2 The Range of Health Research

- Evaluating the impact of health policies on health outcomes
- Developing and testing new interventions for preventing or treating illness

■ 1.2 The Goal of Health Research

The goal of population-focused health research as a whole is to make discoveries that can benefit society, such as:

- The identification of emerging or existing health problems that should be addressed
- The testing of new interventions for preventing or treating diseases
- The contribution of information to the scientific literature that researchers and policymakers use when creating new plans and policies
- The synthesis of existing knowledge so that it can be applied by others

The goal of any one research project is usually modest: to contribute a bit of information that, when pooled with other researchers' information, will provide an evidentiary foundation for change. Research is unlikely to make a researcher rich or famous. It does not offer much in the way of instant gratification because it takes months or years to progress from an initial research idea to the dissemination of findings. Even after the findings are published, few studies lead to immediate changes in health status or health practices. Still, the researcher may enjoy many positive outcomes:

- The acquisition of new skills
- The satisfaction of personal curiosity
- The fulfillment of degree or work requirements
- The opportunity to become a published author
- The possibility that, at some point in the future, the researcher's work will contribute in at least some small way to making at least one person healthier (FIGURE 1-3)

This last outcome describes the fundamental reason for conducting health research.

Societal Benefits	Personal Benefits
• Identification of health concerns and/or methods for promoting health and preventing disease and disability	• Attainment of new knowledge by systematically investigating a topic
• Acquisition of evidence for improving clinical and public health practices and policies	• Development and/or refinement of a new skill set (and possible fulfillment of the requirements of an educational program or employer)
• Expansion of the scientific literature that sets the foundation for future research, policies, and practices	• Satisfaction of exploring an area of interest and seeing a project through to completion

FIGURE 1-3 Societal and Personal Benefits of Health Research

Health research is not a value-neutral activity. Many health scientists are passionate about promoting health and preventing disease in individuals and populations. Health research does not require detachment from the topic under investigation. Health researchers may appropriately express an enthusiasm for making new discoveries and for helping people. Personal passion can be reflected in the chosen research topics and in the way research is conducted—in study designs, in interactions with research participants, and even in the careful analysis of data and written reports.

This is not to say that values trump science. Health scientists must demonstrate respect for those who might be impacted by their research in at least several very important ways. They must conduct methodologically sound, scientifically rigorous, and culturally appropriate research. Also, they must honestly report the methods used and the results observed, even if the results are not the ones they had hoped for at the start of the study. Because personal values and professional ethics are such an integral part of health research, this book incorporates the themes of research ethics and virtues into all its parts. The book does not confine these themes to the specific chapters on research ethics and research ethics committees.

Anyone who is committed to seeing a new and valid project through to completion can contribute to advancing health science. Health research does not require a license. It does not require a doctorate or a master's degree. It does not even require coursework in research methods, although that is certainly helpful. The best way to learn about health research is to do actual research and to learn firsthand how the research process works and what it requires:

- Patience
- Carefulness
- Attention to detail
- Perseverance

- The willingness to learn all the background knowlegde and skills that are required
- The ability to criticize and revise one's own work and writing

■ 1.3 The Research Process

This book is intended to serve as a handbook for population health researchers. The chapters are organized according to the five steps of the research process. Regardless of the goals of a research project or the approach for achieving them, the steps are pretty much the same (FIGURE 1-4). First, identify a study question, and, second, select a general study approach. These two steps require a back-and-forth mind-set because the approach selected may require the refinement of the study question. Once the objectives and approach are set, the last three steps are to design the study and collect data, to analyze the data, and to write a report about the findings. These steps apply to every health research project, whether it is an investigation of an outbreak of gastroenteritis following a company picnic in London, a systematic review of the published literature intended to identify environmental risk factors associated with cataracts, or the analysis of data from thousands of participants in a drug trial.

This guidebook is not meant to be a compendium of everything that health researchers know about study design, data collection, and statistical analysis. Instead, it provides a comprehensive overview of the entire process. As a research project unfolds, most researchers benefit from consulting specialized references. These references can take the form either of advanced textbooks and other library resources or of human experts: professors, supervisors, colleagues, coauthors, librarians, statistical consultants, and others. Chapter 5 provides some suggestions on how to assemble a research support team. Also, many excellent books and online resources contain the advanced technical information required for complex study designs and analytic techniques.

Health research is both a scientific and a social process. Most research projects necessitate many, many hours of independent (and often isolated) work. However, health research, at its core, is about health-related issues affecting individuals and communities—issues that cannot be addressed in isolation. Health scientists communicate with one another primarily through published articles and, to a lesser degree, via presentations at professional conferences. Research that is not published or disseminated in some way will never shape the policies and practices that make people healthier. Thus, every

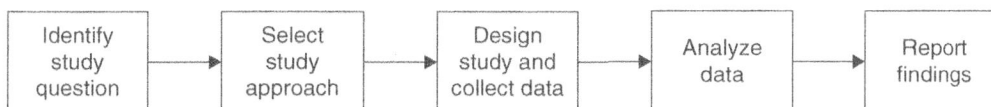

FIGURE 1-4 **The Research Process**

person initiating a new research project should write up the results and consider submitting them to a professional journal for consideration. This is not to say that all research will be published. Publication depends on:

- The appropriateness of the research topic for a wide audience
- How well designed the study is and whether it uses valid methods
- How compelling and well written the manuscript is

The final section of this book provides tips about writing and editing strategies, as well as a step-by-step guide for preparing a manuscript for review and publication. If the goal is to publish the findings of a study—and it often should be—then the researcher must prepare for publication at every step of the process.

Identifying a Study Question

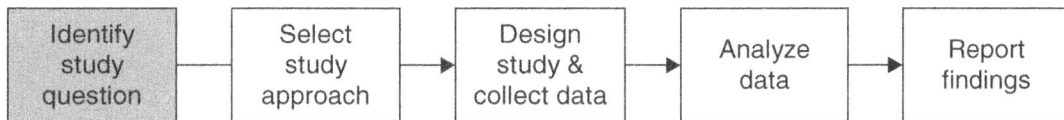

| Identify study question | → | Select study approach | → | Design study & collect data | → | Analyze data | → | Report findings |

The first step in the research process is selecting the topic to be the focus of the study. This section describes how to select a general topic, review the literature, focus the scope of the project, and assemble a research support team.

- Selecting a general topic
- Reviewing the literature
- Focusing the research question
- Assembling a support team

Selecting a General Topic

Identifying one workable study topic is perhaps the most challenging part of a research project. Each of the countless possible study topics has its own set of virtues and shortcomings. Topic selection is one of the few steps in research in which creativity is not just allowed but required. Although study design, data collection, and data analysis must all follow a restrictive set of accepted methods, picking a study topic calls for the expression of personal interests.

▦ 2.1 Brainstorming and Topic Mapping

A brainstorming session can be a good starting point for identifying a research topic. Use the categories in FIGURE 2-1 to identify areas of personal interest. Spend a day, several days, or even weeks jotting down possible research areas. Check with friends and colleagues about their ideas. Search abstract databases, and skim journals and books for ideas about potential research themes.

The goal is to create a list of possible research topics and to make it as long as possible. This is not the stage for eliminating ideas because they do not appear feasible. Think big! The ideas do not need to be well formed. Begin by simply listing several diseases or population groups that might be interesting to study. Do some research areas show up several times on the list and appear to be a central theme? Can those topics be grouped or mapped? (It may be helpful to use circles and arrows to visibly group related topics to clarify the connections.) Which broad areas might be enjoyable to explore?

Area	Questions
Values	• What are my interests and personal values? • What research topics are personally meaningful? • Have some understudied conditions that I could explore significantly affected me, my family, or my friends? • Have certain health issues sparked my passion because they reflect what I consider to be an injustice?
Skills	• What knowledge and skills do I already have?
Personal growth	• What new skills do I want to develop?
Connections	• What source populations and/or data sources might be available to me through professors, supervisors, colleagues, and other personal and professional contacts?
Job and/or course requirements	• What does my supervisor or professor want me to study?
Gaps in the literature	• What information is not currently available that would make a contribution to the discipline and/or to improving health practices or policies? (See Chapter 3 for information about how to conduct a literature search.)

FIGURE 2-1 **Brainstorming Questions**

■ 2.2 Key Words

The next step is to refine the areas of interest that were identified through brainstorming. A helpful approach is to compile a list of related keywords. Jot down a long list of words that may help focus the research question. For example, a person who identifies an interest in child health in Africa during brainstorming might then list words like "malaria . . . children . . . Africa . . . bednets . . . Uganda . . . measles . . . vaccination . . . preschool children . . . malnutrition . . . vitamin A deficiency." A person who identifies an interest in aging might list words like "osteoporosis . . . falls . . . bedsores . . . physical therapy . . . calcium . . . bone density . . . making homes safe . . . rehabilitation . . . prevention." The goal is to identify a wide range of specific potential study themes within the major area of interest.

The MeSH (*Medical Subject Headings*) database, developed by the U.S. National Library of Medicine, can be helpful in narrowing the scope of a research area and in identifying the full extent of a research area. Suppose, for example, that a potential area of interest is infection. The MeSH database suggests a variety of narrower topics related to infection, such as cardiovascular infections, sepsis, infectious skin diseases, and wound infection. Within the category of skin diseases, the MeSH database lists a variety of narrower topics, such as cellulitis, dermatomycoses (fungal skin infections), and bacterial skin diseases. Within the category of dermatomycoses, the MeSH database lists yet narrower topics, such as blastomycosis, cutaneous candidiasis, and tinea. Within these categories, MeSH offers even more refined points and still more refined points within successive subcategories.

Searching through the MeSH database can help a researcher in several ways. The researcher can move from a vague interest in infections or skin infections to a more focused interest in, say, fungal skin infections or, even more specifically, ringworm infections. Alternatively, the MeSH database can be used to search for broader or related study ideas. A search for pre-eclampsia, for example, shows that pre-eclampsia is a type of pregnancy complication. It is related to other forms of pregnancy-induced hypertension, such as HELLP syndrome, which may be an equally interesting study topic.

Once a list of keywords has been compiled, the researcher looks for the themes that emerge from them. Can any topics be easily eliminated because they do not fit the researcher's personal interests (Figure 2-1)? Are some keywords particularly interesting?

■ 2.3 Exposure, Disease, Population

Once several possible themes have been identified, each should be refined. Most topics in population health research can be expressed in terms of the following formula: [exposure] and [disease/outcome] in [population]. *Exposures* (FIGURE 2-2) and *diseases* (FIGURE 2-3) can encompass a wide variety of characteristics, some of which are:

- Social and environmental indicators
- Nutritional status
- Infections

Socioeconomic Status	Health-Related Behaviors	Health Status	Environmental Exposures
• Income	• Dietary practices	• Nutritional status	• Drinking water
• Wealth	• Exercise habits	• Immune status	• Pollution
• Educational level	• Alcohol use	• Genetics	• Radiation
• Occupation	• Tobacco use	• Stress	• Noise
• Age	• Sexual practices	• Anatomy and	• Altitude
• Sex/gender	• Contraceptive use	anatomical defects	• Humidity
• Race/ethnicity	• Hygiene practices	• Reproductive history	• Season
• Nationality	• Religious practices	• Comorbidities	• Natural disasters
• Immigration status	• Use of health-care	(existing health	• Population density
• Marital status	services	problems)	• Travel

FIGURE 2-2 Examples of Types of Exposures

Injuries	Communicable/ Infectious Diseases	Noncommunicable/ Chronic Diseases	Neuropsychiatric Disorders
• Bone fractures • Burns • Crush injuries • Frostbite • Gunshot wounds • Near drownings • Poisonings	• Candidiasis • Cholera • *E. coli* • Hookworm • Malaria • Syphilis • Tuberculosis	• Asthma • Cancers • Cataracts • Diabetes • Hypertension • Osteoporosis • Stroke	• Alzheimer's and other dementias • Autism • Depressive disorders • Post-traumatic stress disorder • Schizophrenia

FIGURE 2-3 Examples of Types of Diseases

- Chronic diseases
- Mental health status
- Quality-of-life measures
- Health service use

The *population* is the group of individuals, communities, or organizations to be examined (FIGURE 2-4). The keywords compiled in the previous step often fit into these exposure, disease, and population categories.

The researcher should divide these keywords into three separate lists:

- One for exposures or categories of exposure
- One for diseases or outcomes
- One for specific populations

These exposures, diseases/outcomes, and populations can then be combined to form study questions. For example:

- Are exercise habits [exposure] related to the risk of bone fractures [disease] in adults with diabetes [population]?

- Australian children younger than 5 years old
- Women living in rural Ontario
- Adults with diabetes
- Teachers with at least 10 years of classroom experience
- Individuals newly diagnosed with influenza at St. Mary's Hospital in Newcastle
- Nongovernmental organizations working on issues related to HIV/AIDS in Uganda

FIGURE 2-4 Examples of Types of Populations

- Is reproductive history [exposure] related to the risk of stroke [disease] among women living in rural Ontario [population]?
- Is household wealth [exposure] related to the risk of hospitalization for asthma [disease] in Australian children younger than 5 years old [population]?

The next step is to conduct a review of the existing literature related to a limited number of potential research questions. The list might consist of perhaps 3 to 5 statements in the standard format: [exposure] and [disease/outcome] in [population]. The aim is to identify what is already known about the topic and to determine what new information a new study could contribute.

Reviewing the Literature

Once a general research area has been identified, the next step is to do background reading about the topic. Usually, researchers start with informal sources that provide basic information about the disease of interest, then move on to more formal reports as the aim and scope of the research idea are refined. This process, as a whole, is called "reviewing the literature."

■ 3.1 Factsheets, Websites, and Informal Sources

A starting point for learning about the primary area of interest is to search the Internet for basic background information. Many major public health organizations, such as the World Health Organization (WHO) and the U.S. Centers for Disease Control and Prevention (CDC), have fact sheets about various diseases and risk factors for disease. National governments and international governmental organizations (like the United Nations) also have factsheets, brochures, and websites that provide basic demographic, political, economic, geographic, and other health-related information about countries and regions. Newspapers and popular magazines may also have compelling nontechnical articles about exposures, diseases, and/or populations that highlight what is interesting and important to know about a topic. The websites of disease advocacy organizations, personal websites, and other media may also be helpful in identifying and refining an important and meaningful study question.

However, researchers must be cautious about claims that contradict more formal sources of information. Sources that independent referees do not peer-review may be a helpful as start-up sources of background reading for exploring areas of interest. They are usually not appropriate citations in formal research reports.

■ 3.2 Statistical Reports

When defining specific exposures, diseases, and/or populations of interest, it may be helpful to identify relevant statistics, such as the estimated prevalence of the exposure in a world region, the annual global incidence of a disease, or the size of a particular population.

- For regional- and country-level population measures and comparisons, the World Bank's world development indicators database provides country-reported information about a wide range of topics.
- Additional statistical estimates can be found in the annexes of the annual reports issued by United Nations agencies, like the World Health Organization (*World Health Report*), UNDP (*Human Development Report*), and UNICEF (*State of the World's Children*).
- The annual reports of private organizations, like the Population Reference Bureau and the American Cancer Society, include up-to-date statistical estimates and projections.
- For information about states, provinces, counties, and other smaller governmental units, contact the relevant public health departments.
- The best place to find very specific information about health-related exposures and diseases may be in published scientific articles.

Although statistics may be readily found on the Internet, few are supported by citations and information about who collected the original data, how information was collected, and even when it was collected. When possible, trace the statistic back to its original source rather than relying on second-hand reports. If the source of data is not clear, the statistic may not be trustworthy.

■ 3.3 Abstract Databases

An *abstract* is a paragraph-length summary of an article, chapter, or book. *Health science abstracts* usually provide a brief description of the study population (such as the sample size and the study site), the study design, and the key findings of the study. *Abstract databases* allow researchers to sort through thousands of abstracts for keywords or other search terms. A careful and comprehensive search of at least one major abstract database is the most important component of a careful literature search.

Many health abstract databases are available from libraries via subscription, like CINAHL (Cumulative Index to Nursing and Allied Health), Embase, ISI Web of Science, MEDLINE, and PsycINFO. The most important publicly available health science database is PubMed, which provides access to more than 15 million abstracts (most of which are from MEDLINE). PubMed can be searched with keywords or MeSH terms, using Boolean operators like AND, OR, and NOT. Limits can be set so that results include only abstracts with certain publication years, languages, or other selected parameters. PubMed can also be searched for abstracts by article title, author (using a last name and first initials format, such as "Baker JD" or "Patel AR"), journal, and/or publication year.

A rigorous review process is used to decide which journals are listed in MEDLINE, and not all journals apply for inclusion or are accepted if they apply. (The list of indexed journals is available online.) As a result, there are many peer-reviewed journals that are not included in the MEDLINE or PubMed databases. Therefore, a supplemental search, by means of a general search engine like Google Scholar, may be helpful in identifying additional relevant abstracts. A supplemental search is especially important when the topic of interest is narrow enough to yield only a small or moderate number of hits. Another benefit of these search engines is that they can provide links to the full-text versions of publicly available articles.

■ 3.4 Full-Text Articles

Abstracts provide a glimpse into the content of an article. However, the only way to truly understand a study is to read the full text of the article. Some articles are available online in their entirety as open access articles on journal websites, in digital archives like PubMed Central, or on the personal websites of the authors themselves. Most university libraries subscribe to hundreds or thousands of online journals that allow patrons to access electronic versions of articles. Most university libraries also have a limited number of journals available in print form on their shelves, but a physical search of the stacks is unlikely to be required unless the article is relatively old. Universities often offer free or low-cost interlibrary loan services to affiliates. "Loans" of journal articles usually take the form of electronic files or photocopies of the article that need not be returned.

When none of these options results in a copy of the article of interest, a final option is to contact the author directly and ask for a copy. Many PubMed entries include the e-mail addresses for article authors, and many journals provide contact information along with the abstract for the articles on their websites. At minimum, PubMed entries and most journal articles list the institutional affiliations of authors, and an Internet search for those institutions will often yield contact information. Most researchers are flattered that someone is interested in their work; there is no risk in asking. At worst, the researcher will get no response to the request. At best, the author might send an electronic copy of the article and an offer of further assistance within minutes of the request.

Once the researcher acquires a copy of the full-text article, a practical plan of action is to:

- Re-read the abstract.
- Look carefully at the tables and figures, because the most important results are usually displayed in the tables or figures.
- Then read (or at least skim) the entire text of the article.

It may also be useful to take notes about which exposures, diseases, and populations the study examined and how they all relate to the proposed new research project. Additionally, a thorough review of the reference lists of the most relevant articles is needed to ensure that all of the critical works in the area of research have been identified.

■ 3.5 What Makes Research Original?

Every researcher is looking for an "original" topic. This can be a paralyzing prospect for anyone who thinks that originality requires the discovery of a newly emergent disease in a previously unrecognized people group on a remote island. Such remarkable discoveries are occasionally featured in the news, but the vast majority of original research is far less dramatic. For a research project to be considered original, it needs to have only one substantive difference from previous work. That could be a new exposure of interest, a new disease of interest, a new source population, a new time period under study, or a new perspective on a field of exploration.

FIGURE 3-1 illustrates this point. An original research project could look at a new potential risk factor (E_2) for a disease (D_1) that is already well studied in a population (P_1). It could look at whether an exposure (E_1) that is known to increase the risk of one disease (D_1) in a population (P_1) also increases the risk of a second disease (D_2). Or it could see whether the association between an exposure (E_1) and a disease (D_1) observed in one or more parts of the world (P_1 and P_2) is also true in another part of the world (P_3). Or a research project could aim to synthesize everything that has already been published on the association between an exposure (E_1) and an outcome (D_1) by doing a thorough literature review.

For example, a literature review might find that several studies have shown that older adults (the population) who take 30-minute walks several times a week (the exposure) score higher on memory tests (the disease or outcome) than adults who do not routinely walk for exercise. A proposed new study could examine:

- Whether playing table tennis (a new exposure) is equally effective at improving memory in older adults (the same disease and population)
- Whether older adults who walk several times a week (the same exposure and population) also improve their balance (a new disease or outcome)
- Whether walking improves memory (the same exposure and disease) in children (a new population)

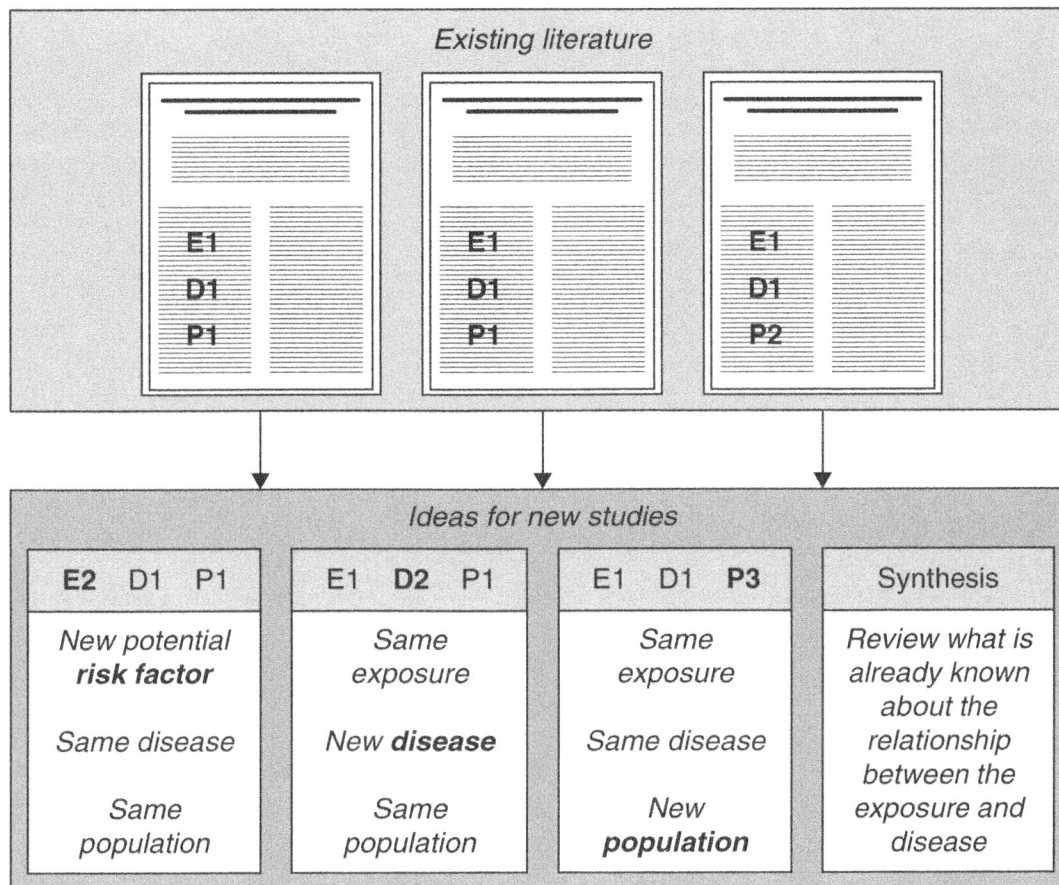

FIGURE 3-1 Ideas for New Studies

Having identified a new study idea, the researcher must conduct a further, thorough review of the literature to confirm that the area has not already been examined.

Thus, the real challenge in reviewing the literature and selecting a study question is not finding a previously unexplored topic. The main challenge is to limit the research project to one solid idea out of the many possibilities. Very few studies create whole new areas of research. The goal of nearly every research project is to contribute an incremental step forward within an area of research. The aim is to find and address *gaps in the literature* (that is, missing pieces of information that a new study could fill) and to build on previous work.

Focusing the Research Question

After identifying a general research topic, the researcher needs to develop a specific and workable research question.

■ 4.1 Study Approach

The decision about the exact study question must be made in conjunction with the decision about the study approach to use. At a minimum, a choice must be made early in the research process about how the new data will be collected (FIGURE 4-1):

- *Primary study:* The data will be collected from individuals.
- *Secondary study:* An existing data set will be analyzed, or data extracted from existing records will be statistically analyzed.
- *Tertiary study:* The existing literature will be reviewed.

Research Approach	Study Plan
Primary	Collect and analyze new data
Secondary	Analyze existing data
Tertiary	Review and synthesize the literature

FIGURE 4-1 Primary, Secondary, and Tertiary Research

Study Approach	Key Questions to Ask
• Collection and analysis of new data	• What are possible source populations? • Will it be possible to recruit enough participants?
• Analysis of existing data	• What are possible sources of usable data files? • What questions can be explored with the available data?
• Review of the literature	• Does the researcher have access to adequate library resources? • Can the researcher reasonably expect to acquire *all* of the needed articles?

FIGURE 4-2 **Key Considerations**

Each of these three major study approaches has its own critical considerations (FIGURE 4-2).

- If new data will be collected, the researcher has great freedom in selecting study topics but may be restricted by the ability to recruit adequate numbers of participants. (Chapters 16 and 17 explain why sample size is important and how to estimate whether a sample size will be adequate.)
- If existing data will be analyzed, then a data file (or another source of data, such as existing patient records) must be identified. The researcher must also be prepared to select a study question based on the content of the data file and on the variables in the data set that others have not already explored.
- If the plan is to synthesize current knowledge by conducting a literature review, the researcher must be prepared to track down the full text of all relevant articles. Researchers with a university affiliation need to check with the university library about its policies (and possible fees) for acquiring articles that are not part of the university's collections. Researchers without a university affiliation must consider the costs involved in accessing all of the required articles.

■ 4.2 Study Goal and Specific Objectives

The literature review and consideration of a study approach should lead to the selection of one very specific study topic that can be stated in terms of a single overarching study goal or study question. FIGURE 4-3 lists several types of common study goals in the health sciences. A *study goal* often includes the specific exposure, disease, and population that will be the focus of the study.

After finalizing the overarching study goal, the researcher should identify three or more *specific objectives, aims, or hypotheses* that stem from the main study goal. Each

- To describe the incidence or prevalence of a particular exposure or disease in one well-defined population
- To assess the perceived health-related needs of a community
- To compare the levels of exposure or disease in two or more populations
- To identify possible risk factors for a particular disease in a population
- To test the effectiveness of a new diagnostic or assessment method or of a new therapy or treatment
- To evaluate whether an intervention shown to be successful in one population is equally successful in a second population
- To examine the impact of a program or policy
- To synthesize or integrate existing knowledge

FIGURE 4-3 Examples of Study Goals

of these specific objectives should take the form of a measurable question or a "to" statement, either of which uses action verbs. Each should represent a logical step toward answering the main study question. For example, the study goal may be "to assess the impact of lead poisoning on school performance in kindergarten students in southeast Michigan." The three specific objectives for this study may be:

1. To measure the prevalence of high blood lead levels in a random sample of kindergarten students in southeast Michigan
2. To determine whether children in that sample with high blood lead levels have lower scores on academic tests than children with lower blood lead levels
3. To estimate the total impact of high blood lead levels on kindergarten performance in southeast Michigan by applying the rates in the sample population to the total population of the region

All three of these specific objectives relate to the overall goal of the study and provide a clear pathway for achieving the main goal. Most published scientific papers list the study goal and specific objectives in the last paragraph of the introduction section. The specific aims of already published papers related to the topic are often helpful resources when refining the research objectives of a new study.

■ 4.3 Checklist for Success

A consideration when narrowing the focus and clarifying the aims of a new research project is the likelihood that the project can actually be successfully completed. FIGURE 4-4 summarizes some of the critical questions to ask before committing to a particular project.

Area	Questions
Purpose and significance	• What will the study contribute? • What will be new and noteworthy about the study? • Can the importance and necessity of this project be justified? • How will the study enhance the body of knowledge in its discipline? • Who will benefit from the study besides the researcher? • How will the study help individuals and/or communities live healthier lives? • How might the study contribute to improving health practices and/or policies?
Scope and feasibility	• Is the scope of the intended project reasonable and manageable—neither too broad nor too narrow? • Can the proposed study question actually be answered? • Can the researcher answer the proposed study question?
Capacity and collaborators	• Does the researcher have the knowledge and skills needed to conduct the study? • Does the researcher have access to collaborators who have the expertise needed for the project? (See Chapter 5 for information on assembling a support team.)
Money and materials	• Are there adequate financial resources to conduct the study? • Does the researcher have access to equipment, space, and other physical requirements? • Given the resources available, can the researcher reasonably expect to conduct a scientifically rigorous and valid study?
Time	• Does the researcher have the time to conduct this study? • Does the researcher have the time to make this an excellent study that does not waste health resources?
Population or data	• If the plan is to collect new data from individuals, does the researcher have access to a reasonable source population and an adequate number of participants? • If the plan is to analyze existing data or to write a review paper, does the researcher have access to a reasonable existing data set and/or to an extensive library collection?
Ethics	• Will the researcher be making good use of the resources available? • Has the researcher considered the relevant ethical issues, especially those related to the collection and use of individual-level data? (See Chapter 21 for the ethical issues that should be considered.) • Is the researcher prepared to conduct culturally appropriate and scientifically rigorous research?
Target audience	• Who is likely to be interested in the findings? • Is the resulting paper likely to be publishable?

FIGURE 4-4 Questions Essential to the Success of the Project

Assembling a Support Team

Research projects benefit from the input of technical and cultural experts. Researchers should assemble a team of collaborators early in the research process.

■ 5.1 Collaborators, Consultants, and Friends

Scientific research is rarely completed by one person working alone. Although some papers in the health sciences have solo authors, most papers have about four coauthors, and some have dozens of coauthors. Thus most projects are headed by a lead researcher, defined here as the researcher who will do the majority of the work. (Sometimes the term *lead researcher* is instead used to refer to the *senior researcher*, an experienced researcher who guides the work of a newer investigator.) Once the lead researcher has committed to doing a research project, it is helpful to assemble a support team (FIGURE 5-1).

Some of the support team members will be core collaborators and coauthors of the resulting report. They might include:

- A supervisor or other experienced researcher who serves as a mentor and advisor during the research process
- An expert on the research topic or the study population
- An expert on the study design or other methods being used for the research
- A statistician

Core collaborators			Additional technical support		Personal support
Lead researcher	Advisor/ mentor/ supervisor	Study design/ statistics expert	Librarian	Statistician	Friends and family
Subject matter expert	Cultural expert	Other key contributors	Laboratory technician	Other technical experts	Co-workers and/or classmates

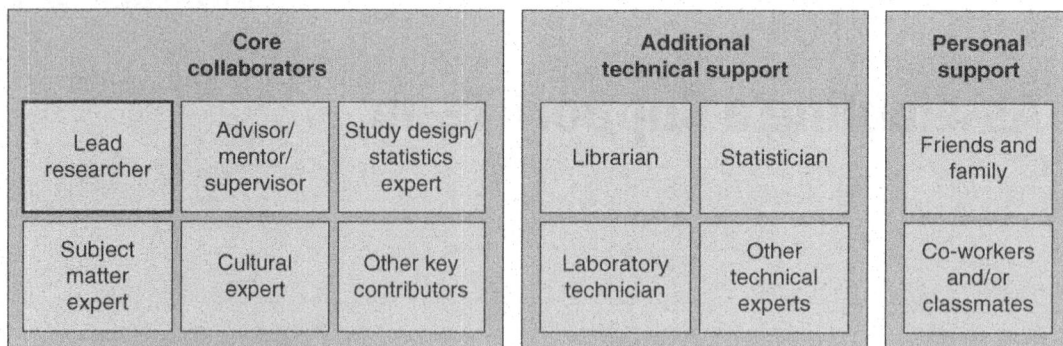

FIGURE 5-1 Support Team Members

- Other key contributors who are significantly involved in the design and conduct of the study and in the editing and polishing of the manuscript

For international research projects, at least one local researcher should be a coinvestigator who is involved in every step of the research process, including the identification of the study question, the design of the study, and the collection of data.

Additionally, the study may require the help of still others. The researcher might have to consult with technicians who will contribute to the project on a very limited basis and who may not meet the criteria for being coauthors. Before these potential contributors spend time on the project, be sure to have a conversation with them about their expectations regarding authorship. For example, a statistical consultant either may prefer to be paid for an hour helping a researcher think through analytic options or may request authorship in return for the development of a data analysis plan. Keep track of all the librarians, statistical consultants, laboratory technicians, and other experts and consultants who contribute to the project. Be sure to thank them in the acknowledgments section of any manuscript that benefitted from their contributions.

The final important group of supporters consists of the family members and friends who care more about the researcher than about the research. Additionally, a researcher might want to join a writing group or a research support group made up of other new researchers who will be able to offer advice and motivation along the way.

■ 5.2 Authorship Criteria

The International Committee of Medical Journal Editors (ICMJE) has established criteria for authorship in the health sciences that most journals in the field have adopted. According to the criteria listed in ICMJE's Uniform Requirements for Manuscripts

Submitted to Biomedical Journals, each coauthor must have met *all three* of the following conditions:

- Substantial contributions to conception and design *and/or* acquisition of data *and/or* analysis and interpretation of data
- Drafting the article *and/or* revising it critically for important intellectual content
- Final approval of the version to be published

The guidelines specifically add that "acquisition of funding, collection of data, or general supervision of the research group alone does not constitute authorship." People who provide funding and supervision for a project may qualify for authorship, but that criterion alone is not sufficient. Just like any other contributor, sponsors and supervisors must make a meaningful intellectual contribution to a project to merit authorship.

A contributor does not have to engage in all parts of the study—designing the study *and* collecting the data *and* analyzing it—to be a coauthor. Participating in a meaningful way in any one of these parts of the study fulfills the first condition. However, participating in design, conduct, and analysis is not sufficient to earn authorship. Authorship requires participation in the writing of the research report. The second ICMJE authorship condition is that all coauthors must make a consequential intellectual contribution to the written product stemming from the research project, either by drafting part of the manuscript or by critically revising it. The third condition is intended to ensure that persons are not listed as authors against their will or without their knowledge. A manuscript should not be sent to a journal until all the coauthors have consented to the submission.

According to these guidelines, as examples:

- A person who conducts interviews for the project but does not contribute further would not be eligible for authorship. However, an interviewer who also writes a paragraph for the discussion section would meet authorship criteria.
- A hospital laboratory technician who analyzes blood samples of patients included in a clinical study but makes no further contributions would not be eligible for authorship. A lab tech who analyzes the samples and writes part of the methods section describing laboratory techniques would be a coauthor.
- A data entry assistant who makes no additional contributions to the project would not be considered an author. A data manager who runs statistical tests and creates a table for the manuscript would meet authorship criteria.
- A technical editor who cleans up the grammar and spelling in a manuscript does not earn authorship. An editor who raises important questions about the interpretation of the results and the meaning of the work may be eligible for authorship.

The intention is that "all persons designated as authors should qualify for authorship, and all those who qualify should be listed." There should be no so-called *gift authorships*, in which someone is given honorary coauthorship without having significantly contributed to the work. Conversely, there should be no *ghost authorships*, in which someone who has made a substantial intellectual contribution is not appropriately recognized.

■ 5.3 Authorship Order

For most disciplines in the health sciences, the *first author* (or *lead author*) is the person who was the most involved in writing the manuscript. Although this is often the person who took the lead in the whole study process from design through analysis and writing, this is not always the case. Sometimes the person who designed the study and collected the data is unable to conduct the analysis and to write up the results, or that person (often a senior researcher) turns the responsibility of writing the manuscript over to someone else who is subsequently listed as the first author. Sometimes multiple people are involved in study design and data acquisition, and one person is asked by the group to take the initiative to generate a draft paper. Sometimes organizations make data sets available to researchers for analysis; they do not request authorship for any of the employees involved in study design or data collection because none of them are involved in writing the manuscript. In all of these situations, the person who does most of the writing is often designated as the first author. When there is any doubt as to who is making the most significant contribution, the decision about who will be first author should be made in consultation with all of the people who took a major role in conducting the study.

The remaining authors are usually listed in order of contribution, which is usually defined in terms of time dedicated to the project as well as intellectual contribution. The person who contributes the second most amount of time and energy to the project is listed as second author, and so on. When many coauthors are involved, it is sometimes difficult to quantify the relative contributions of, say, the seventh and eighth authors. In this situation, the coauthors should be consulted about their preferences, but the best solution may be to list authors with equal contributions in alphabetical order.

The one exception to the rule about listing authors in order of contribution is that the senior author is often listed last, unless he or she has contributed significantly to the project and prefers to be listed in another position based on the level of contribution. Not every paper has a senior author. However, students are usually required to have a professor or other approved supervisor oversee their work. It is usually helpful for a relatively inexperienced researcher to seek out a mature investigator to serve as the senior author on the paper. The senior author may or may not be heavily involved in the day-to-day details of the study but meets the authorship criteria by providing clarity and direction along the way and by providing critical feedback on the manuscript. Additionally, the senior author can serve as a mediator if disputes about authorship or other issues arise. An experienced researcher will be able to provide insight into disciplinary standards and can prevent or resolve many of the issues that might befuddle a newer researcher.

■ 5.4 Decisions About Authorship

Sometimes, determining whether a person has made important intellectual contributions to a project is challenging. In such cases, it is helpful to decide ahead of time, in consultation with each potential contributor, the role each person will play. At the end of the project, there should be no surprises about who is being included or excluded as an author. Check with each interviewer, each laboratory technician, and each data manager and supervisor about expectations. Have this conversation *before* any of them begins work on project-related tasks. If everyone agrees that a person making a minor contribution will not be a coauthor, make sure that the person is not asked to write any part of the paper or to provide critical feedback on a draft. If everyone agrees that someone will be a coauthor, make sure that the person has the opportunity to make an important intellectual contribution to the paper.

Decisions about who will be listed as a coauthor on a report, poster, or paper, as well as the order in which those persons will be listed, should be made as early as possible in the research process. Publications are an important metric of success in the sciences and academia, and authorship is often the only reward for the time put into a project. As a result, authorship decisions can be very stressful. They can trigger strong emotional responses, and they can sometimes even harm relationships among researchers. Lead researchers therefore need to be transparent with everyone involved in the project not only about who will and will not be contributing in ways that merit coauthorship, but also about the role each person will be playing. A growing number of journals now require a description of what each coauthor contributed and how each met authorship criteria. It might be helpful to draft that statement *before* writing any other part of the paper so that anyone who sees the draft knows what is expected of each coauthor.

Sometimes, the list of expected contributors might change during the project. Perhaps a new collaborator is needed to run advanced statistics or to provide an expert's perspective on the policy implications of the work. In such cases, all coauthors need to be immediately informed about the addition. Sometimes, the addition of new collaborators significantly alters another contributor's position in the order of authors, perhaps bumping a person from second to fourth author. Then the affected person must be consulted and an agreement reached before any promises are made to the new coauthors.

Any disputes over authorship criteria or the order of authors are usually best referred to the senior author on the paper. Also helpful are the accepted guidelines for authorship from ICMJE, a professional society, or the target journal.

Selecting a Study Approach

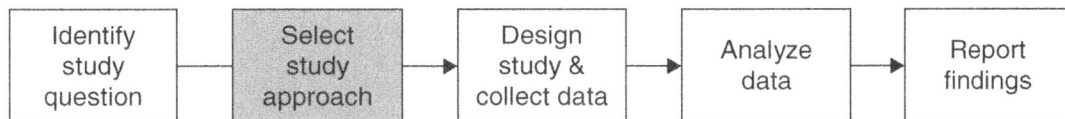

STEP

2

Identify study question	Select study approach	Design study & collect data	Analyze data	Report findings

The second step in the research process is to select a general study approach. This section provides an overview of 8 common study designs.

- Reviews or meta-analyses
- Correlational (ecological) studies
- Case series
- Cross-sectional surveys
- Case control studies
- Cohort studies
- Experimental studies
- Qualitative studies

Overview of Study Approaches

There are many good study designs for population health research. This chapter is an overview of the eight most common ones.

■ 6.1 Types of Study Approaches

Eight study approaches, as listed in FIGURE 6-1, will be discussed in detail in the following chapters. The figure does not represent a comprehensive list of all type of studies. Many studies use variations of one of these approaches, and in other studies a hybrid of two approaches might be suitable. This book covers a wide range of study approaches, including the collection and analysis of new data, the analysis of existing data, and reviews of the literature, because all of them are valid and helpful research methods in the health sciences.

The approach selected must be appropriate for the goals of the study. For example, if the goal is to see whether an intervention is effective, an experimental design is likely to be the only suitable one. If the goal is to understand populations, to describe patterns, or to ask research questions that are not focused on causality, the best design may be an observational one, such as a cross-sectional or cohort study. Often the best study approach is the analysis of existing statistical data rather than the collection of new data from individual participants. Sometimes the best approach is a systematic review

Study Approach	Goal
Review/meta-analysis	Synthesize existing knowledge
Correlational (ecological) study	Compare average levels of exposure and disease in several populations
Case series	Describe a group of individuals with a disease
Cross-sectional survey	Describe exposure and/or disease status in a population
Case-control study	Compare exposure histories in people with disease (cases) and people without diseases (controls)
Cohort study	Compare rates of new (incident) disease in people with different exposure histories or follow a population forward in time to look for incident diseases
Experimental study	Compare outcomes in participants assigned to an intervention or control group
Qualitative study	Seek to understand how individuals and communities perceive and make sense of the world and their experiences

FIGURE 6-1 **Summary of Study Approaches**

or meta-analysis. Sometimes several different study approaches can be appropriate for exploring the relationship between an exposure and a disease. In these situations, it is helpful to consider several other factors, including the availability of existing data, the expected duration of the study, and the populations available for inclusion in the study.

◼ 6.2 Primary, Secondary, and Tertiary Studies

A first critical decision is whether to collect new data from individuals (a primary analysis), use existing data (a secondary analysis), or write a review article (a tertiary analysis). (See FIGURE 6-2.) Primary studies are often time-consuming because they require the collection of new data from participants. However, primary studies also give the researcher control over items like the selection of a source population and the content and wording of the questionnaire. The obvious advantage of secondary and tertiary analyses is that a researcher may be able to move fairly quickly from the definition of the study question to the analysis of related data. However, only a limited number of data sets and publications are available for analysis. Also, they might not include either the exact variables or the population of greatest interest to the researcher.

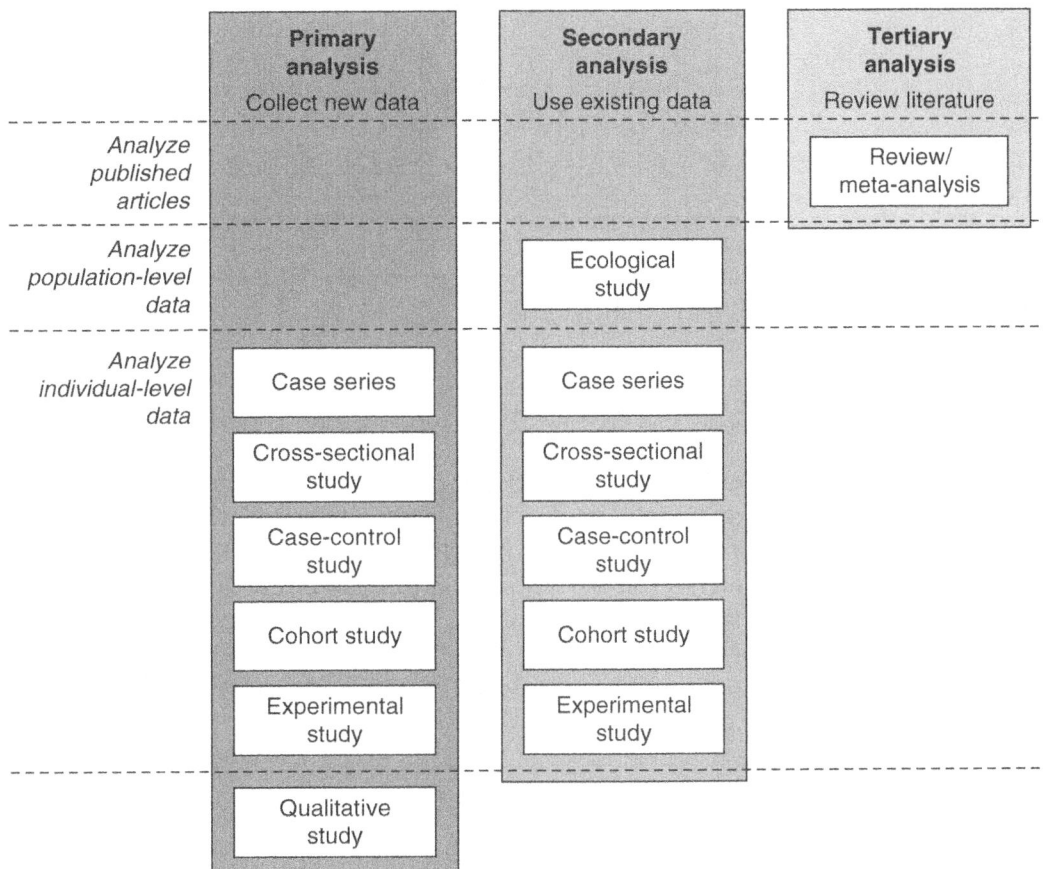

	Primary analysis Collect new data	Secondary analysis Use existing data	Tertiary analysis Review literature
Analyze published articles			Review/meta-analysis
Analyze population-level data		Ecological study	
Analyze individual-level data	Case series	Case series	
	Cross-sectional study	Cross-sectional study	
	Case-control study	Case-control study	
	Cohort study	Cohort study	
	Experimental study	Experimental study	
	Qualitative study		

FIGURE 6-2 Primary, Secondary, and Tertiary Study Approaches

■ 6.3 Study Duration

The time required for collecting and analyzing data varies from study to study. Some primary studies call for the collection of all needed information from participants at one point in time. Others require participants to be followed for weeks, months, or even years (FIGURE 6-3). The timeline for a secondary study might be very short if an entire data file can be downloaded from a website. On the other hand, secondary data collection might become labor-intensive if old hospital charts have to be retrieved, read, coded, and entered into a database. The duration of tertiary studies is highly dependent on library access and on the number of publications that need to be acquired, read, and summarized.

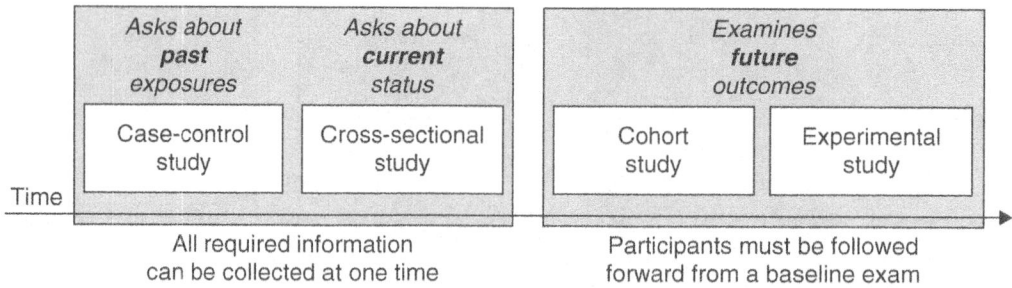

FIGURE 6-3 Time Frame for Primary Data Collection

■ 6.4 Primary Focus: Exposure, Disease, or Population?

Every study approach is oriented toward a particular kind of population (FIGURE 6-4). For example, case series and case-control studies both focus on individuals with a particular disease, while many cohort studies focus on individuals with a particular exposure. Cross-sectional studies seek to recruit a study population that is representative of a well-defined larger population. Researchers who have relatively easy access to a population of interest, such as a group of individuals with a particular disease or exposure, often choose a study approach based on its appropriateness for the available participants.

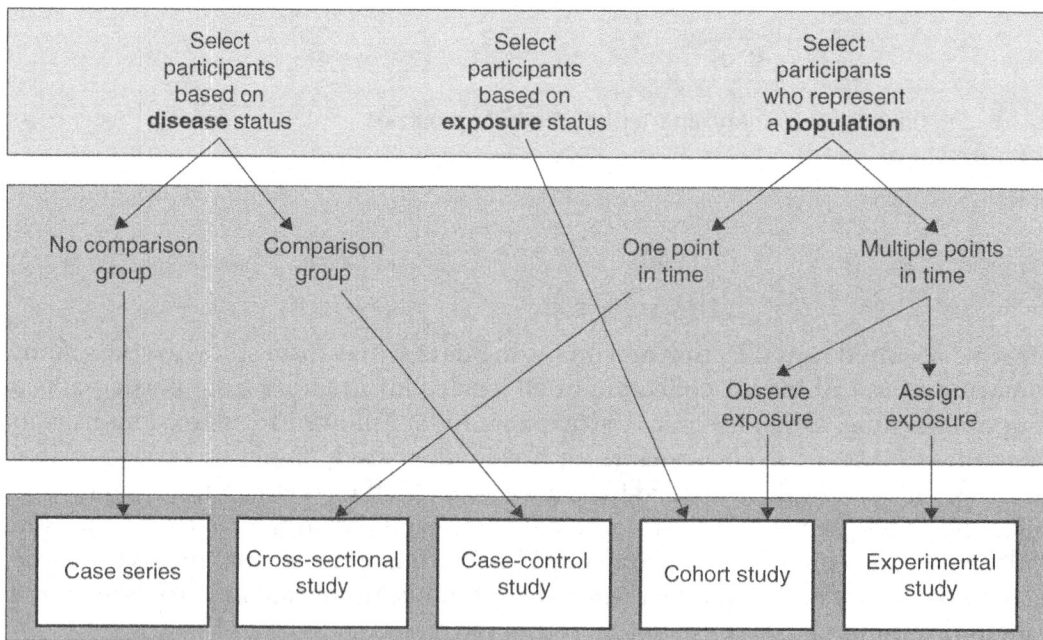

FIGURE 6-4 Population Selection for Each Study Approach

Reviews

Either a systematic review of the literature or a meta-analysis can be used to carefully gather all prior publications on a specific topic and summarize them to provide a big-picture analysis.

Approach	Narrative Review	Systematic Review	Meta-Analysis
Objective	Synthesize existing knowledge	Synthesize existing knowledge	Synthesize existing knowledge
Primary study question	What conclusions about this topic are supported by previous studies?	When all previously published studies on this topic are examined, what conclusions can be drawn?	When the results of all previously published studies on this topic are merged, what is the summary statistic?
Population	Published literature	Published literature	Published literature
When to use the approach	The goal is to describe a new perspective on a topic that can be supported by the existing literature.	The goal is to compare the findings of previous studies on a well-defined topic.	The goal is to summarize previous findings using pooled statistics.

FIGURE 7-1 Key Characteristics of Reviews and Meta-Analyses

Approach	Narrative Review	Systematic Review	Meta-Analysis
Requirements	The researcher has excellent library access.	The researcher has excellent library access.	The researcher has excellent library access.
	The researcher has a unique perspective on the topic.	The researcher can obtain every relevant article.	The researcher has strong quantitative skills.
First steps	1. Decide what story the article will tell.	1. Decide on the specific objectives of the review. 2. Select the search methods that will be used to find potentially relevant articles. 3. Select inclusion and exclusion criteria for articles.	1. Decide on the specific objectives of the review. 2. Select the search methods that will be used to find potentially relevant articles. 3. Select the inclusion and exclusion criteria for the articles. 4. Decide how to assess the quality of the studies. 5. Decide how the results of the studies will be combined into one summary statistic.
What to watch out for	Limited publication venues	Publication bias	Studies that cannot be fairly compared
Key statistical measure	No statistics are required.	No statistics are required, but providing some results from included studies may be helpful.	Summary measures for included studies must be reported.

FIGURE 7-1 (continued)

■ 7.1 Overview

Although much scientific research is about the identification of something new, the goal of a review article is to engage in the scholarship of integration: to synthesize what is already known about a topic by connecting previous studies and offering new interpretations of their contributions to scientific knowledge. A review article in the health sciences requires:

- An extensive search of the literature
- The extraction of key information from relevant articles
- The clear and concise presentation of this information

Writing a review article—whether a narrative review, systematic review, or meta-analysis (FIGURE 7-1)—is a way to become an expert in the literature on a well-defined topic. This outcome is a good one in and of itself, but it can also be a helpful step in preparing for future primary or secondary analyses. Well-written and comprehensive review articles often become foundational for new research in the field because they summarize what is already known about an area of inquiry. Review articles are often cited more often than reports of individual field studies because they synthesize the content from many original research articles.

However, review articles have limitations. Not all journals publish review articles (especially reviews that the editors do not solicit). So their likelihood of publication may be lower than that of other study approaches. A good review requires meticulous library work, followed by the careful compilation and interpretation of information. Yet reviews are sometimes perceived to be a less rigorous form of research than projects that collect new data and/or involve statistical analysis. They are therefore sometimes regarded as having less worth than other types of research.

■ 7.2 Selecting a Topic

When starting a review article, the most important decision is to select a topic that is narrow enough that all the relevant publications can be acquired. The topic may need to be modified after a preliminary search, depending on the number of articles available. If a search of an abstract database yields only 8 articles, the topic probably needs to be expanded; if a search produces 352 articles, the topic needs to be narrowed to a more specific disease condition, to a smaller geographic area, or to a reduced scope.

For example, a review of risk factors for cardiovascular disease would be cumbersome. A very long book would be required in order to cover all the identified risk factors. An article-length manuscript would provide such a superficial level of information that it would not be a true review. There is a greater likelihood of success for a review article on, say, obesity and the risk of hypertension in second-generation Japanese Americans or on tobacco use and the risk of atrial fibrillation in postmenopausal women. Thus, the reviewer benefits by limiting the types of risk factors, the particular cardiovascular diseases, and the population groups that will be examined.

■ 7.3 Library Access

No review article can be written without excellent library access because *every* relevant article must be identified and obtained. This usually requires access to a university library that allows patrons to make numerous interlibrary loan requests. Before starting a review project, a researcher should check with a university librarian regarding the library's policies and the fees that patrons may have to pay for the use of interlibrary loan services. The researcher must also maintain a meticulous system for tracking articles that have already been acquired, those that have been requested but not yet received, and those that need to be requested.

■ 7.4 Narrative Reviews

Narrative reviews tell a story about a topic using evidence from the literature to support the "plot." A narrative review might summarize critical clinical aspects of a disease, present an epidemiological profile for a disease, or propose a new theory. Because they are intended to convey a perspective and not merely compile facts, narrative reviews must be carefully organized by theme, methodology, chronology, or some other guiding principle.

Narrative reviews are becoming less common as readers and editors push for the use of systematic methods. This means that researchers must be prepared to justify their selection of this approach. A narrative review works best when the researcher has a unique perspective on a topic or a particular expertise in the field that can be drawn on without using a systematic search strategy. A narrative is also appropriate when the researcher has developed a unique organizing framework.

■ 7.5 Systematic Reviews

Systematic reviews use a fixed method to select relevant articles. This process is designed to minimize the bias that might occur when review article authors handpick the articles they want to highlight. Therefore, after the identification of the study question, the most important decision in a systematic review is the selection of keywords and inclusion criteria. The goal is to craft a search strategy that identifies all the articles ever published on the narrow, well-defined area covered by the review. Once the articles are identified from one or more abstract databases, each article is screened to see whether it is eligible for inclusion. Relevant information is extracted from all eligible articles and presented in table form. Then the trends and key observations are summarized. Chapter 24 provides a more detailed description of the systematic review process.

■ 7.6 Meta-Analysis

The goal of a *meta-analysis* is to combine the results of several high-quality articles that used similar methods to collect and analyze data into one summary statistic. After the study question has been defined, meta-analysis usually begins with a comprehensive systematic review of the literature to identify every single possibly relevant article. Each of these articles is read to ensure that it meets the inclusion criteria, which are usually more restrictive than they are for systematic reviews. These restrictions are important because a summary statistic is only meaningful when every study included in the meta-analysis has very similar definitions for exposures and outcomes, similar study designs and methods, and similar populations. Trying to combine dissimilar studies could hide real and meaningful differences among populations.

The steps of a meta-analysis are to:

- Use a systematic search strategy to identify relevant articles
- Carefully read each study
- Assess the quality and comparability of each study
- Extract statistical results from each study that meets all inclusion criteria for the meta-analysis
- Combine these statistical results into one summary statistic

The summary statistic should adjust for the varying sample sizes and confidence intervals of the contributing statistical measures. Chapter 24 provides additional information about meta-analysis.

Correlational (Ecological) Studies

A correlational (ecological) study uses population-level data to examine the relationship between exposure rates and disease rates.

Objective	Compare average levels of exposure and disease in several populations
Primary study question	Do populations with a higher rate of exposure have a higher rate of disease?
Population	Existing population-level data are used; there are no individual participants.
When to use this approach	The aim is to explore possible associations between an exposure and a disease using population-level data.
Requirement	The topic has not been previously explored using individual-level data.
First steps	1. Select the sources of data that will be used. 2. Decide on the variables to include in the analysis.
What to watch out for	The ecological fallacy
	Limited publication venues
Key statistical measure	Correlation

FIGURE 8-1 Key Characteristics of Correlational (Ecological) Studies

■ 8.1 Overview

- Does the percentage of adults with multiple sclerosis tend to be higher in countries farther from the equator?
- Does the prevalence of diabetes tend to be higher in provinces with a higher prevalence of obesity?
- Does the rate of asthma tend to be higher in cities with higher levels of air pollution?

Each of these questions can be explored with a correlational study. Also called an "ecological study" or "aggregate study," a *correlational study* uses population-level data to look for associations between two or more group characteristics (FIGURE 8-1).

Because existing data sources are almost always used for correlational studies, the key to success is identifying a data source that contains comparable information about the variables of interest. Information about all the variables of interest must be available for a suitable number of populations, which can be grouped by place or time. For example, place-based populations could consist of all member nations of the United Nations, all 50 states from the United States, the largest 20 metropolitan areas in the United Kingdom, all the counties in the state of Michigan, or a random sample of census tracts in New York City. Time-based studies could use historical data for the past several decades from one or more place-based populations.

■ 8.2 Data for Correlational Studies

For most studies, at least one characteristic of the populations being examined is designated as an *exposure*, and at least one is designated as an *outcome* or disease. Most exposures and outcomes used in correlational studies are in the form of aggregate data, such as the proportion of each population with a particular characteristic or the average value of the variable in the population. For example, the exposure may be the percentage of adults age 30 and older who have not completed at least 12 years of education, the mean income in the population, or the median age. Alternatively, an exposure variable may represent an environmental measure that is likely to be fairly consistent across an entire population, such as the number of rainy days over a given year or the average ultraviolet radiation index during midday in the hottest month of the year. The disease may be measured as, for example, the prevalence of obesity among adults or the annual mortality rate from asthma.

Before conducting a statistical analysis of ecological data, the data must be entered into a spreadsheet. Each population should be assigned to its own row in the spreadsheet. Each exposure and outcome should be assigned to its own column. The data should be filled into the cells in each column so that they line up with the correct population. (See FIGURE 8-2 for a sample data table.)

Population	Exposure 1	Outcome 1
A	48.2	14.1
B	65.1	17.0
C	37.8	14.9

FIGURE 8-2 **Sample Data Table**

The analysis will be valid only if the data points are comparable. If multiple sources of data are used or if the data were collected over a lengthy period of time, then the definition of exposure or disease may differ from one population to another. In some populations, exposures and diseases may be routinely undercounted or routinely over-diagnosed, compared to other populations. Because of the potential lack of comparability, researchers should interpret ecologic associations conservatively.

■ 8.3 Analysis: Correlation

On a scatterplot used to illustrate correlation, each point represents one population in the study. The exposure is plotted on the *x*-axis, and the outcome or disease is plotted on the *y*-axis (FIGURE 8-3).

- When all the points fall neatly in a line, then the correlation is strong.
- When the points are not exactly linear but a line for trend can be drawn, then the correlation is mild or moderate.
- When the points appear to be randomly placed and no obvious line can be drawn through them, then the correlation is weak or nonexistent.
- If higher levels of exposure are linked to higher rates of disease, then the slope is positive.
- If higher levels of exposure are linked to lower rates of disease, then the slope is negative.

For continuous variables and other variables with responses that can be plotted on a number line, a Pearson correlation coefficient (r) should be used to calculate the correlation. For variables that assign a rank to responses or that have ordered categories, use the Spearman rank-order correlation (designated by the letter r or the Greek letter ρ [rho] in most statistical programs). For both tests, the value of r ranges from -1, when all points lie perfectly on a line with a negative slope, to 1, when all points lie perfectly on a line with a positive slope. When $r = 0$, there is no association between the exposure and outcome. (Chapter 27 explains the difference between *parametric tests* like the Pearson correlation and *nonparametric tests* like the Spearman

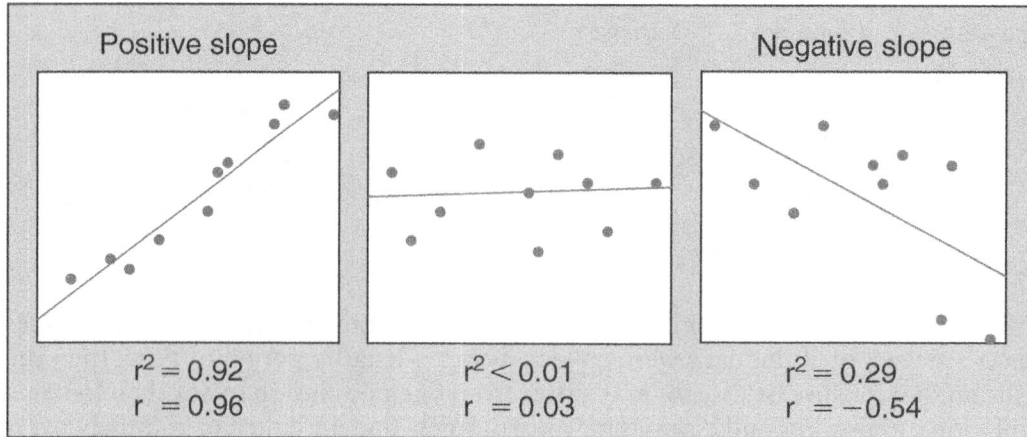

Positive slope

Negative slope

$r^2 = 0.92$
$r = 0.96$

$r^2 < 0.01$
$r = 0.03$

$r^2 = 0.29$
$r = -0.54$

FIGURE 8-3 Correlation

rank-order correlation and Kendall's rank correlation, which is often designated with the Greek letter τ [tau].)

The association between two or more variables can also be reported as r^2, which shows how strong a correlation is without indicating the direction of the association. The value of r^2 ranges from 0 for no correlation to 1 for perfect correlation.

Sometimes more than two variables are being compared or the goal is to understand the relationship between two variables while controlling or adjusting for the effects of other variables. In such cases, linear regression models are used to assess the associations (see Chapter 28).

Note that a measure of correlation is different from a test for intercorrelation. A test for *intercorrelation* examines whether two or more related variables that are part of a survey instrument measure various aspects of the same thing. For example, Cronbach's alpha and the Kuder-Richardson Formula 20 (KR-20) are measures of internal consistency among items on a questionnaire. Tests of intercorrelation examine the reliability of survey instruments and are not the same as tests of correlation that compare two or more independent variables. For ecological studies, correlation, not intercorrelation, should be assessed.

■ 8.4 Age Adjustment

Sometimes the populations being compared have very different age structures. For example, one or more populations might skew considerably younger or older than the others. If so, age adjustment may be necessary to make a fair comparison among populations. *Direct age adjustment* requires knowing the exposure and/or disease rates by age group in each population. These rates are then applied to a standardized population, and a summary age-adjusted population rate is calculated for each population being compared. *Indirect age adjustment* methods can sometimes be used to compare populations for which age distributions are known but age-specific rates of exposure and/or disease are not known.

■ 8.5 Avoiding the Ecological Fallacy

Correlational studies compare groups rather than individuals. No individual-level data are included in the analysis, only population-level data. The incorrect attribution of population-level associations to individuals is called the *ecological fallacy*, and this error should be avoided. Even though a *population* with a higher rate of exposure to something has a higher rate of disease than populations with lower exposure rates, *individuals* in that population who have a high level of exposure do not necessarily have the disease. The experience of an individual in a population may vary significantly from the population average. For example, it would be incorrect to assume that any one individual from a country with a high average body mass index (BMI) will be obese or that an individual from a country with a low average BMI will not be obese. However, it is appropriate to identify trends in populations and to use those observations to generate hypotheses for individual-level studies that will test for relationships between the characteristics of interest in individuals. Correlational studies are a useful starting point for generating hypotheses about associations, but they are not the final word on risk factors for disease.

CHAPTER 9

Case Series

A case report describes one patient. A case series describes two or more patients who have the same disease condition or who have undergone the same procedure.

Objective	Describe a group of individuals with a disease
Primary study question	What are the key characteristics of the cases in this study population?
Population	All individuals in the study must have the same disease or be undergoing the same procedure.
When to use this approach	A source of cases is available, and no comparison group is required or available.
Requirement	An appropriate source of cases is available.
First steps	1. Specify what new and important information the analysis will provide. 2. Identify a source of cases. 3. Assign a case definition. 4. Decide on the characteristics of the study population that will be described.
What to watch out for	A lack of generalizability
Key statistical measure	Only descriptive statistics are required.

FIGURE 9-1 Key Characteristics of a Case Series

◼ 9.1 Overview

A *case series* describes a group of individuals with a particular disease (FIGURE 9-1). A case series is possible only when a researcher has access to an appropriate source of cases and when there is a compelling reason to write about those cases. This study approach can be useful for:

- Describing the characteristics of and similarities among a group of individuals with the same signs and/or symptoms of disease
- Identifying new syndromes and refining case definitions
- Clarifying typical disease progression
- Developing hypotheses for future research

Some case series for rare conditions may require only a handful of participants. Others may include several hundred individuals.

◼ 9.2 Case Definitions

A researcher conducting a case series must select one disease of interest, determine what will be new and interesting about the study, and identify an appropriate and

Category	Example 1	Example 2
Disease/procedure	Whooping cough (ICD-10 code A37)	Liver transplantation
Person	Any person with a confirmed case of whooping cough, defined as an acute cough of any duration with isolation of *Bordatella pertussis* from a clinical specimen *or* a cough lasting 2 or more weeks with paroxysms of coughing, inspiratory "whoop," or post-tussive vomiting and contact with a laboratory-confirmed case of pertussis	Adult patients (ages 18 and older at the time of transplant), excluding those who were not receiving their first liver transplant and those who received multi-organ transplants
Place	Residents of Big City whose diagnoses were reported to the Big City Health Department (which requires notification of all diagnoses of pertussis)	Patients who had transplant surgery at the Oakville Regional University Medical Center
Time	First sought clinical care between January 1 and March 31, 2011	Recipients of liver transplants between January 1, 2000, and December 31, 2008, who were followed for a minimum of 2 years post-transplant

FIGURE 9-2 Sample Case Definitions

available source of cases. The next step is to establish a clear case definition that spells out inclusion and exclusion criteria. Participants may be selected from clinical locations that use ICD codes (i.e., diagnoses based on the International Classification of Diseases, known more formally as the International Statistical Classification of Diseases and Related Health Problems). If so, the ICD number can be part of the case definition, but a code alone is rarely sufficient to cover all inclusion and exclusion criteria. A more comprehensive case definition will include a disease description plus any relevant person, place, and time characteristics (FIGURE 9-2). Case definitions are also essential for any outbreak investigation, no matter which study approach is used to investigate the epidemic.

■ 9.3 Special Considerations

A case series might involve primary data acquired by interviewing cases about their experiences using a questionnaire and/or qualitative techniques. The data might be supplemented or confirmed with a review of the participants' medical records. Alternatively, a case series can be (and often is) based solely on secondary data, usually acquired from a review of patient charts.

When medical records will be consulted as part of the data collection process, it is often helpful to create a questionnaire that guides the extraction of information from medical records. One of the limitations of relying on patient charts is that they usually contain only information deemed at the time of examination to be clinically relevant. The medical information in patient files is not recorded for research purposes, so records are unlikely to contain all the information that researchers would like to know. Less relevant signs and symptoms, patient comments, and clinician observations are usually not recorded. As a result, the absence of a specific note about a symptom or history does not necessarily mean that the exposure was not present, just that it was not recorded. A data extraction tool should include space to indicate the absence of a desired piece of information in the record. During the analysis and interpretation stage of the research project, the researcher should carefully consider the amount and type of missing information.

Case series come with special requirements. All case series studies require approval by a research ethics committee, as well as informed consent from participants and/or the careful use of existing records. Case series researchers must pay special attention to protecting the identities of participants. This is especially important when the disease or procedure is relatively rare and/or when the place and time characteristics are so narrow that individuals familiar with the source community might be able to recognize the participants. In most situations, all potentially identifiable information must be removed prior to publication. For example, an image should not contain any identifying marks that could reveal the participant's identity. (In some situations, patients may be allowed to give permission for potentially identifiable information or images to be published.)

■ 9.4 Analysis

Most case studies do not require any numbers beyond simple counts and frequencies, but some may benefit from the use of well-defined measures of morbidity and mortality. For example, the *case fatality rate* is the proportion of persons with a particular disease who die as a result of that condition. (This is different from the *crude mortality rate*, which is the proportion of members of a general population who die of any condition during a specified time period. It is also different from the *proportionate mortality rate*, which is the proportion of deceased members of a population whose death was attributable to a particular cause.) In some situations, comparative statistical tests may be possible when comparing subpopulations within the population of cases or when comparing before-and-after measures for the same individual participants.

Although many case series do not have any time dimension, some follow patients for days, months, or years. In this type of study approach, the case series becomes, functionally, a cohort study in which all participants are defined by their disease status. Chapter 12 discusses cohort study approaches.

Cross-Sectional Surveys

A cross-sectional survey provides a snapshot of the health status of a population at one point in time. Cross-sectional surveys, sometimes called "prevalence studies," are among the most popular study approaches in the health sciences because they allow for the relatively rapid collection of new data.

Objective	Describe the exposure and/or disease status in a population
Primary study question	What is the prevalence of the exposure and/or disease in the population?
Population	The study participants must be representative of the population from which they were drawn.
When to use this approach	Time is limited and/or the budget is small.
Requirement	The exposures and outcomes are relatively common, and the likelihood of being able to recruit several hundred participants is strong.
First steps	1. Define a source population. 2. Develop a strategy for recruiting a representative sample. 3. Decide on the methods to be used for data collection.
What to watch out for	Nonrepresentativeness of the study population
Key statistical measure	Prevalence

FIGURE 10-1 Key Characteristics of Cross-Sectional Surveys

10.1 Overview

The goal of a *cross-sectional survey*, also called a prevalence study, is to measure the proportion of a population with a particular exposure or disease. This determination should be made at one point in time based on a representative sample of a population. (See FIGURE 10-1.) Cross-sectional surveys are used to:

- Describe communities
- Assess population needs
- Evaluate programs
- Establish baseline data prior to the initiation of longitudinal studies

10.2 Representative Populations

In some ways, cross-sectional studies use the simplest study design. The researcher just asks a few hundred people to complete a short questionnaire and then analyzes the data. However, there is one very important requirement: the participants must be reasonably representative of some larger population. The researchers cannot simply ask friends, the fans attending a youth football game, or individuals attending a chiropractic clinic to complete a survey and then assume that the results of the survey will be generalizable to all town residents. If the results are intended to reflect the profile of an entire town or other population group, then the study's sampling strategy must recruit a population that is as diverse as the town.

Chapter 16 has more detailed information about populations for a cross-sectional survey, and Chapter 17 explains how to estimate sample size requirements.

10.3 Analysis: Prevalence

Cross-sectional surveys measure the prevalence of various demographic characteristics, exposure histories, and disease states in one well-defined population at one point in time. The most common way to report results for a cross-sectional survey is simply to report the prevalence rate, which is the proportion of the population with a given trait at the time of the survey.

Comparative measures can also be used. For example, prevalence ratios compare the prevalence of a characteristic in two population subgroups by taking a ratio of their prevalence rates. Because a cross-sectional survey has no time dimension, it cannot be used to assess causality. An exposure can be said to be "associated" or "related" to a disease, but a cross-sectional survey cannot show that an exposure caused a disease.

Case-Control Studies

A case-control study compares the exposure histories of people with and without a particular disease in order to identify likely risk factors for the disease.

Objective	Compare exposure histories in people with disease (cases) and people without diseases (controls)
Primary study question	Do cases and controls have different exposure histories?
Population	Cases and controls must be similar except for their disease status.
When to use this approach	The disease is relatively uncommon, but a source of cases is available.
Requirement	A source of cases is available.
First steps	1. Identify a source of cases. 2. Assign a case definition. 3. Decide what type of control population will be appropriate for the study. 4. Decide whether cases and controls will be matched.
What to watch out for	Recall bias
Key statistical measure	Odds ratio (OR)

FIGURE 11-1 Key Characteristics of Case-Control Studies

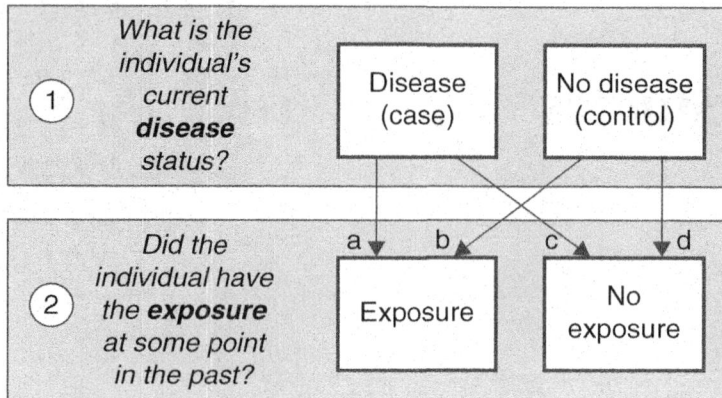

FIGURE 11-2 Framework for a Case-Control Study
(The letters a, b, c, and d correspond to the equation shown in Figure 11-4.)

■ 11.1 Overview

Individual participants in a *case-control study* are selected for inclusion in the study based on their disease status. Participants with the disease of interest are classified as *cases*. Those without the disease are classified as *controls*. Both cases and controls are asked the same set of questions about past exposures (FIGURES 11-1 and 11-2). A case-control study is often the best study approach for identifying risk factors for a disease. This is especially so when the disease is relatively uncommon and a study of the general population is unlikely to yield more than a few cases. A special type of statistic—an odds ratio—is used to identify likely risk factors.

■ 11.2 Finding Cases and Controls

Because case-control studies require a fairly sizable number of cases, the first step is to identify an appropriate and accessible source of individuals with the disease of interest. Hospitals, specialty clinics, physicians' offices, public health agencies, disease registries, and disease support groups may be able to assist researchers in identifying individuals who are likely to meet the study's case definition.

(Regardless of the source, in most situations these organizations will not release any information about individuals until after a research project has received approval from an appropriate ethics oversight committee. When the information is disclosed, the researcher must exercise extreme care to protect the privacy of potential participants and the confidentiality of their personal information.)

Chapter 16 provides additional details about the selection of cases.

All cases must have the same disease, disability, or other health-related condition. So the next step in a case-control study is to develop a working case definition that specifies exactly what characteristics must be present or absent for a person to be deemed a case. Clinical manuals and publications stemming from previous studies of the disease can be helpful references for drafting and refining the inclusion and exclusion criteria. The case definition should include person, place, and time characteristics (see Figure 9-2).

Next, an appropriate source of controls must be selected. Depending on the goals of the study, controls may be recruited from, among other sources:

- Friends and relatives of cases
- Hospital or clinic patients without the disease of interest
- The general population

Controls must be reasonably similar to cases except for their disease status. So the inclusion and exclusion criteria for cases that do not specifically relate to the disease should also apply to controls. For example, if cases must be males between 25 and 39 years of age, controls must also be men in this age group.

Chapter 16 provides additional details about the selection of controls for case-control studies.

■ 11.3 Matching

Early in the design process, a decision must be made about whether to match cases and controls. There are three basic options for *matching*: no matching, frequency (group) matching, and matched-pairs (individual) matching.

Some studies use no matching. They simply assume that similar inclusion and exclusion criteria for cases and controls will result in case and control populations that have similar distributions according to sex, age group, socioeconomic status, and other characteristics.

Some studies use *frequency (group) matching* for a few variables to ensure comparable case and control populations. For example, suppose a study is using hospitalized cases and controls. The researcher may select, for each case, one control from the hospital registration files who was admitted the same week as the case, who is the same sex as the case, and who is within ± 3 years of the age of the case. In addition to identifying only one similar case, frequency matching can be used to identify two, three, or more times as many controls as cases. (Estimating the sample size required for different ratios of cases to controls is described in Chapter 17.) For group matching like this, the goal is to recruit a control population that is similar to the case population. Individual cases are not tied to individual controls during analysis. So the analysis uses the same approaches as those used for unmatched case-control studies.

Some studies use *matched-pairs (individual) matching*. Each case is personally linked to a particular individual control. This approach is fairly common in genetic studies, in which a case is linked to a genetic sibling or other close genetic relative for analysis. This kind of matched-pairs approach requires a special type of analysis that is discussed at the end of this chapter.

For both frequency matching and matched-pairs matching, it is important not to overmatch. The variables used for matching criteria cannot be considered as exposures during analysis. For example, suppose cases and controls are frequency matched based on the date of hospital admission, sex, and age. The case and control populations will likely end up, perhaps artificially, having the same proportion of admissions in April, the same percentage of males, and about the same mean age. As a result of this forced similarity, the study will not be able to examine whether cases are more or less likely than controls to require hospitalization in a certain month, to be males, or to be octogenarians. Additionally, when there are more matching characteristics, it can be difficult to find controls who meet all of the matching criteria.

■ 11.4 Special Considerations

Once the key decisions about study design are made, planning for data collection may begin, as described in the third section of this book. Researchers must keep two special points in mind when designing the survey instrument for case-control studies.

First, in case-control studies, all participants must be asked questions that confirm whether each is a case, a control, or neither. The questions must ensure that only confirmed cases and controls are included in the analysis. Adhering to strict definitions for what constitutes a case and what constitutes a control minimizes the risk of *misclassification bias*.

Second, researchers must be aware of the risk of *recall bias*, which occurs when cases and controls systematically have different memories of the past. This type of risk is particularly important in case-control studies. Participants are often asked to recall distant events from the past that cannot be confirmed by documents from when the exposure would have occurred. Cases may be searching for answers to questions about why they have become ill. As a result, they may have more vivid memories of participation or lack of participation in activities perceived to be risky or beneficial. For example, adult cases in a study of night blindness may report that they rarely ate carrots as children. They may say this not because they never ate carrots but because they assume that, if they had eaten lots of vegetables high in vitamin A when they were kids, they would have had good vision as adults. Alternatively, cases may overestimate childhood carrot intake. They may wonder why they developed night blindness when they have such fond memories of happily munching on carrot sticks every day at lunch in grade school. The reality may be that they ate carrots only once a month. Controls, on the other hand, are unlikely to think much about risk factors for poor eyesight. They may recall eating carrots sometimes rather than rarely or often.

Because of recall bias, this study might find a significant difference in the reported childhood consumption of carrots between cases and controls. This may be the result even if in reality there was no difference in the average diet of the two groups. Alternatively, the survey may fail to capture a true difference in dietary history. Although there is no way to prove that recall bias is occurring, the results of case-control studies must be interpreted cautiously in light of the possibility that differential recall may have influenced the findings.

■ 11.5 Analysis: Odds Ratios

Researchers considering using a case-control study approach must become familiar and comfortable with the concepts of odds and odds ratios. The odds ratio is the measure of association that readers will expect to be reported for a case-control study. *Odds* are the most familiar from their connection with betting. A horse with an equal chance of winning a race (50% likely to win) or of losing a race (50% likely to lose) is said to have "even odds," or odds of 1 (50%/50%). Similarly, a case-control study compares the chance of having had a particular exposure to not having had it (FIGURE 11-3). If 50% of the participants in a study report a history of exposure and 50% report no exposure history, then the odds of exposure are 50%/50%, or 1. If 25% report having the exposure and 75% do not, then the odds are 25%/75%, or 0.33. If 2% report being exposed in the past and 98% report not being exposed, then the odds are 2%/98%, or 0.02.

Case-control studies use, as their main measure of association, the ratio of the odds of exposure in cases to the odds of exposure in controls. This is called an *odds ratio (OR)*. FIGURE 11-4 shows a 2×2 table for a case-control study. Two-by-two tables compare two dichotomous (i.e., yes/no) variables. In the 2×2 table for an unmatched case-control study, the columns are for disease status (case = yes and control = no) and the rows are for exposure status (exposed = yes and not exposed = no). All of the participants in the study are assigned to one of the four resulting boxes: (*a*) cases with an exposure history, (*b*) controls with an exposure history, (*c*) cases with no exposure history, and (*d*) controls with no exposure history. As a check, the total number of cases in the study should be $a + c$, and the total number of controls in the study should be $b + d$.

The odds of exposure in cases are the number of cases with exposure (*a*) divided by the number of cases without the exposure (*c*). The odds of exposure in controls are the number of controls with the exposure (*b*) divided by the number of controls without the exposure (*d*). Simple algebra shows that the equation for the odds ratio of $(a \div c)/(b \div d)$ can be simplified to

$$OR = \frac{ad}{bc}$$

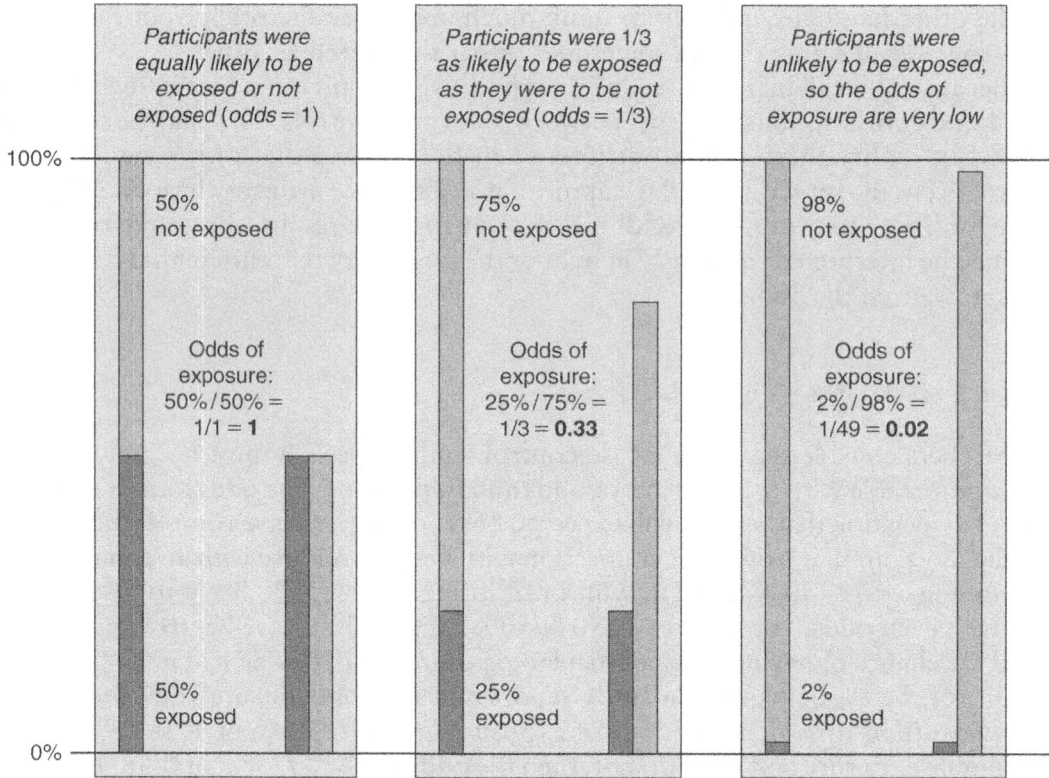

Participants were equally likely to be exposed or not exposed (odds = 1)

100%

50%
not exposed

Odds of
exposure:
50%/50% =
1/1 = **1**

50%
exposed

Participants were 1/3 as likely to be exposed as they were to be not exposed (odds = 1/3)

75%
not exposed

Odds of
exposure:
25%/75% =
1/3 = **0.33**

25%
exposed

Participants were unlikely to be exposed, so the odds of exposure are very low

98%
not exposed

Odds of
exposure:
2%/98% =
1/49 = **0.02**

2%
exposed

0%

FIGURE 11-3 **Odds**

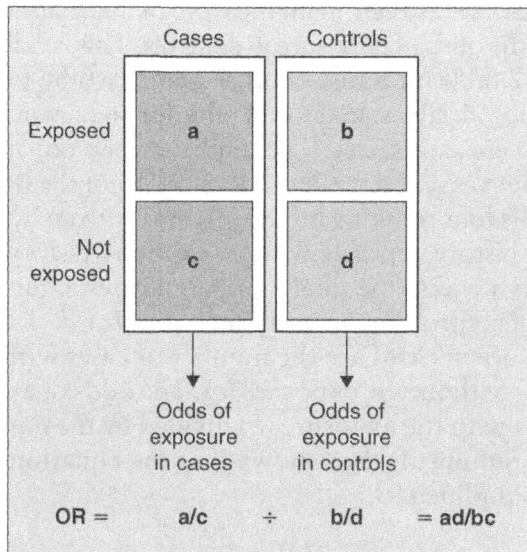

Cases   Controls

Exposed   a   b

Not
exposed   c   d

Odds of   Odds of
exposure   exposure
in cases   in controls

OR =   a/c   ÷   b/d   = ad/bc

FIGURE 11-4 **Odds Ratio (Point Estimate)**

- If the odds of exposure are the same for cases and controls, then OR = 1.
- If the OR is greater than 1, then cases have higher odds of exposure than controls, implying that the exposure was risky.
- If the OR is less than 1, then cases have lower odds of exposure than controls, implying that the exposure was protective.

The 95% confidence interval shows whether an OR is statistically significant (FIGURE 11-5).

- Suppose the 95% confidence interval (95% CI) overlaps OR = 1. This occurs when the lower end of the confidence interval is less than 1, suggesting protection, while the higher end of the confidence interval is greater than 1, suggesting risk. In that situation, the OR is said to be not statistically significant, and the exposure and disease are deemed to have no association.
- If the entire 95% confidence interval is less than 1, then the OR is statistically significant, and the exposure is deemed protective.
- If the entire 95% confidence interval is greater than 1, then the OR is statistically significant, and the exposure is deemed risky.

Computer- and Internet-based statistical programs are available that calculate the point estimate for the OR (the value of ad/bc), along with its corresponding 95% confidence interval, when the values for a, b, c, and d are entered. Sample output is shown in FIGURE 11-6. One example has an odds ratio of 1.588 and a 95% confidence interval of (1.027, 2.453), implying that the exposure was risky. The other example has an odds ratio of 1.158 and a 95% confidence interval of (0.650, 2.066). Since the 95% CI overlaps 1, the association is not statistically significant. The correct conclusion in this example is that there is no association between the exposure and the disease.

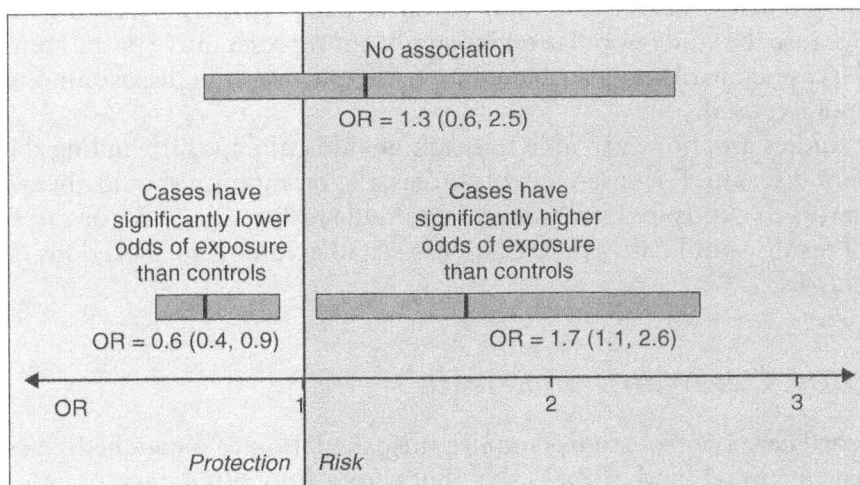

FIGURE 11-5 Interpretation of the Odds Ratio Based on Its 95% Confidence Interval

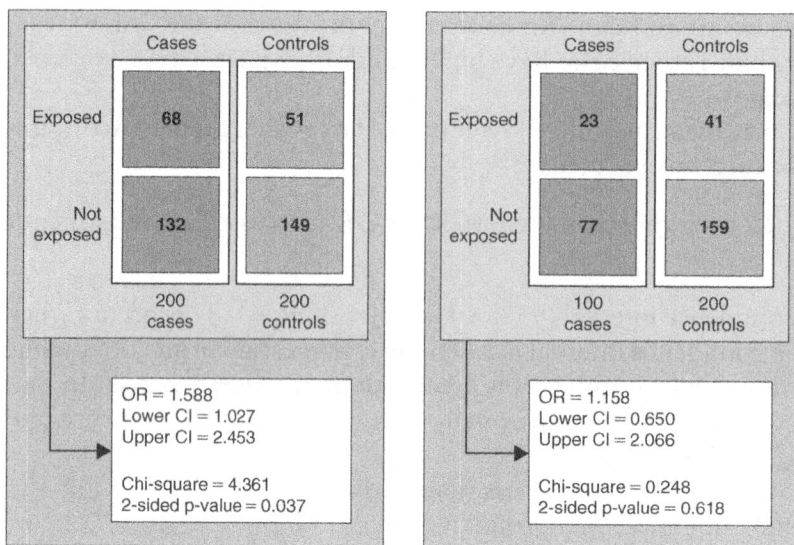

FIGURE 11-6 Examples of Odds Ratio Calculations

For a case-control study, it is incorrect to say that "the exposed had a higher (or lower) rate of disease than the unexposed" because the rates of disease in exposed and unexposed participants are not known. Case-control studies recruit participants because they have or do not have a disease. Usually about 50% of participants in a case-control study are cases even if cases make up less than 1% of the community from which the study population was drawn. As a result, the prevalence of disease among exposed persons *in the study population* could be 70% even when the prevalence of disease among exposed persons *in the community* from which participants were drawn is less than 1%. Because the study population is usually not representative of the community as a whole, case-control studies are unable to calculate rates of disease among the exposed and not exposed.

Case-control studies are, however, able to examine odds of exposure among the diseased and the not diseased. For case-control studies, the orientation should always be from disease status to exposure history, and from odds rather than risks or rates. So the phrasing of results should always be that "cases had greater (or lesser) odds of exposure than controls."

■ 11.6 Matched Case-Control Studies

Individually matched case-control studies require the calculation of a matched-pairs odds ratio that uses a special kind of 2×2 table that shows how often pairs of cases and controls had the same or different exposure histories (FIGURE 11-7). When both the

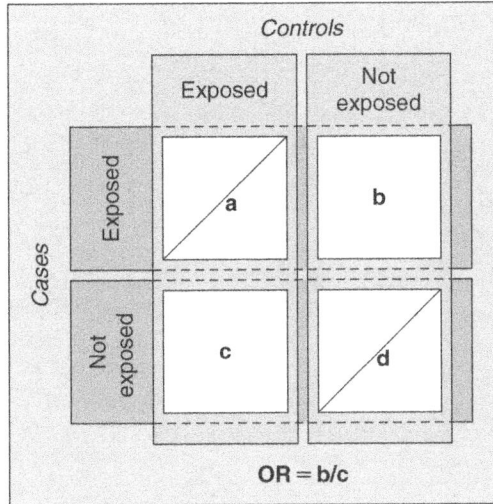

FIGURE 11-7 Matched-Pairs Odds Ratio

case and control in a matched pair have the same history of exposure or no exposure, when their experiences are *concordant* (cells *a* and *d*), they do not provide much useful information about the potential relationship between the exposure and the disease. However, when the exposure histories for a pair are *discordant* (cells *b* and *c*), they provide an indication about whether the exposure is likely to be risky or protective. A ratio of the number of times the case was exposed and the control was not (*b*) to the number of times the control was exposed and the case was not (*c*) provides an estimate for a special type of odds ratio.

- If *b*/*c* is greater than 1 and the 95% confidence interval (calculated using all four categories in the figure, including the concordant pairs) does not overlap 1, then cases are more likely than controls to have been exposed. This implies that the exposure is risky.
- If *b*/*c* is less than 1, and the 95% confidence interval does not overlap 1, then cases were less likely than controls to have had the exposure. This implies that the exposure is protective.
- If the 95% confidence interval includes 1, then there is no association between the disease and the exposure.

For additional information about how to analyze individually matched (matched-pairs) case-control studies, consult a reference that specifically addresses matched-pairs methods and analysis.

Cohort Studies

> *A cohort study follows participants through time to calculate the rate at which new disease occurs and to identify risk factors for the disease.*

Approach	Prospective or Retrospective Cohort	Longitudinal Cohort
Objective	Compare rates of new (incident) disease in people with different exposure histories.	Follow a population forward in time to look for new (incident) diseases.
Primary study question	Is exposure associated with an increased incidence of disease?	Is exposure associated with an increased incidence of disease?
Population	Participants must be similar except for exposure status.	Participants must be available for follow-up months or years after enrollment.
	Because the goal is to look for incident disease, no one can have the disease of interest at the start of the study.	The study participants must be reasonably representative of the population from which they were drawn.
When to use this approach	An exposure is relatively uncommon, but a source of exposed individuals is available.	The goal is to examine multiple exposures and multiple outcomes, and time is not a concern.
Requirements	A source of individuals with the exposure is available.	There is adequate time and money for the study.

FIGURE 12-1 Key Characteristics of Cohort Studies

First steps	1. Identify a source of individuals with the exposure. 2. Decide what type of unexposed individuals will be an appropriate comparison group.	1. Select a source population. 2. Select the exposures and outcomes that will be assessed. 3. Decide how often data will be collected. 4. Develop a strategy for minimizing the burden of participation and maximizing benefits and incentives.
What to watch out for	Participant drop-outs (prospective studies) or missing records (retrospective studies)	Participant drop-outs
	Information bias, in which the exposed participants are more thoroughly examined for disease than unexposed participants	Potential data management challenges if lots of information is collected at many points in time.
Key statistical measure	Relative risk (rate ratio, RR)	Relative risk (rate ratio, RR)

FIGURE 12-1   (continued)

12.1 Overview

A *cohort* is a group of similar people followed through time together. (See FIGURE 12-1.) Health research makes use of several types of cohort-based study approaches. All cohort studies have at least two measurement times:

- An initial survey that determines the baseline exposure and disease status of all participants
- One or more follow-up assessments that determine how many participants have developed a new (incident) disease since the initial examination (FIGURE 12-2)

Because information is collected from individuals at multiple points in time, researchers can know with certainty which exposures were present in individual participants before the onset of new disease. This information allows for the identification of potentially causal exposures.

12.2 Types of Cohort Studies

Cohort studies can come in many forms. For simplicity, this chapter will group cohort study designs into three categories: retrospective, prospective, and longitudinal

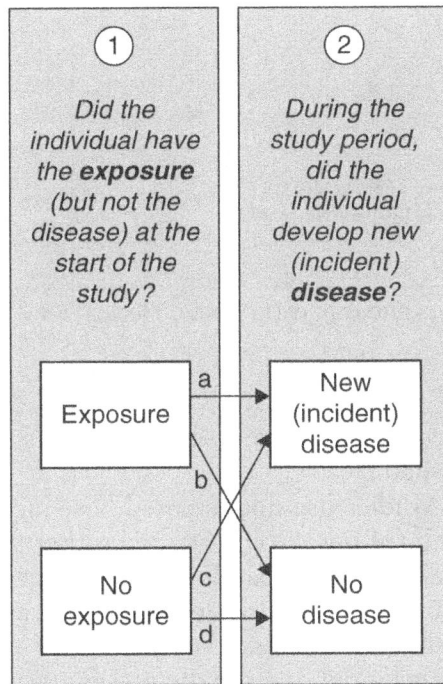

FIGURE 12-2 **Framework for a Cohort Study**

(The letters a, b, c, and d correspond to the equation shown in Figure 12-8.)

(Figure 12-1). Both *retrospective cohort studies* and *prospective cohort studies* recruit participants based on their exposure status. One group of participants is recruited because they are known to have had a particular exposure. A second group is recruited because they are known not to have been exposed. Recruiting based on exposure status makes retrospective and prospective cohort studies the optimal study approaches for uncommon exposures.

The members of the two comparison groups for both types of studies should be similar except for their exposure status. For example:

- A cohort study might compare industrial workers exposed to a certain chemical to workers in a plant that does not use the chemical. It would not be helpful, however, to compare factory workers to office managers.
- A cohort study might compare health outcomes in children with high blood lead levels and low blood lead levels who attend the same elementary school. It would not be as helpful, however, to examine the impact of blood lead levels if the exposed student were from one primary school and the unexposed were from another school. Any differences in health observed might be due to differences in socioeconomic status rather than lead exposure.

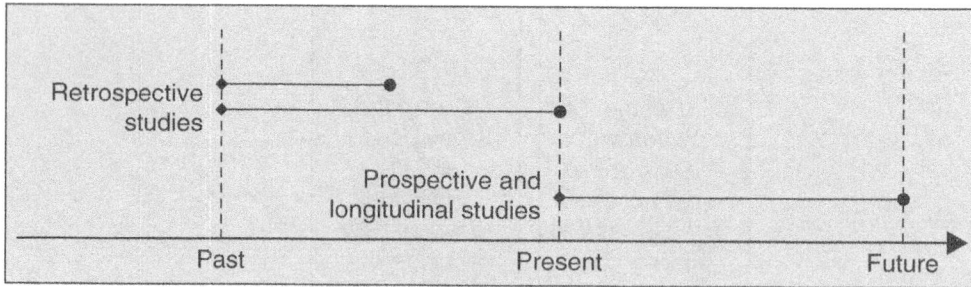

FIGURE 12-3 Times of Baseline and Follow-Up Data Collection for Cohort Studies

The key difference between retrospective and prospective studies is when the baseline measurements are established (FIGURE 12-3).

Retrospective cohort studies use documented baseline information collected at some point in the past and follow the cohort to another point in the past or to the present. Retrospective studies establish baseline information from birth records, school records, medical files, occupational records, or other sources that may be decades old. Then the researcher matches the baseline records to later files or to information solicited directly from the same individuals in the present. For example, a retrospective cohort study might track down two groups of young adults in equal numbers: those born at a particular hospital in a particular year who had low birthweights and those born in the same hospital in the same year who had normal birthweights. The aim could be to see how birthweight influenced adult health status. Similarly, a retrospective study might track down the causes of death after retirement from the armed services for soldiers whose military records indicate whether they served or did not serve in a particular deployment zone.

Prospective cohort studies have a different time orientation. Prospective studies collect baseline data about exposures and outcomes in the present and follow the cohort to some point in the future.

Because all cohort studies examine incident disease, retrospective and prospective studies must be able to demonstrate that the outcome of interest was not present in any members of the cohort at baseline. A retrospective cohort study that looks at the causes of death after the baseline assessment will have no trouble proving that the outcome—death—was not present at the time of the initial assessment. It is more challenging to conduct a retrospective study when the outcome of interest is a condition that may have been present at baseline but not documented.

Longitudinal cohort studies follow a group of individuals forward in time but do not recruit them based on exposure status. Instead, participants are recruited based on membership in a well-defined source population. Longitudinal cohorts may follow all the residents of one town, a representative sample of members of one professional organization, or a cohort of students recruited from the same university.

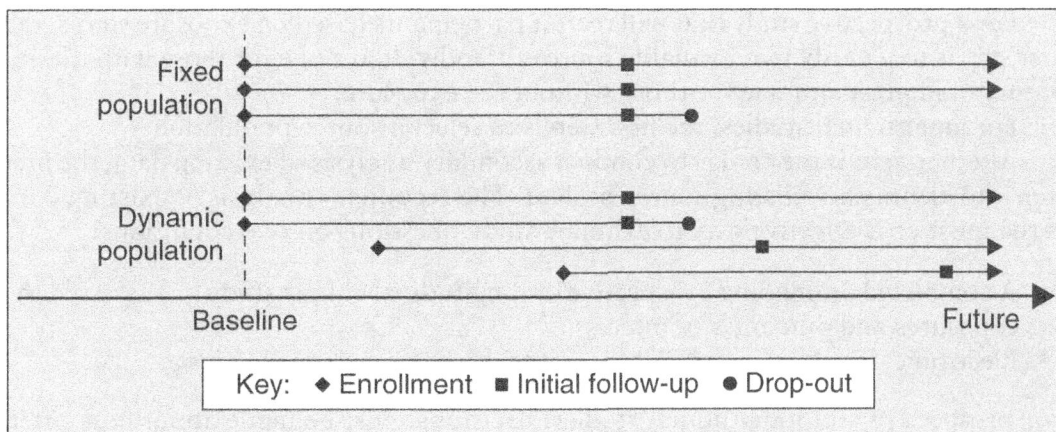

FIGURE 12-4 **Longitudinal Studies**

Individual participants are assessed at baseline for several exposures and diseases. Then they are followed forward in time to determine the incidence rate for one or more outcomes of interest. Longitudinal studies may use a *fixed population* in which all participants start the study at the same time and no one is allowed to join later. Alternatively, they may use a *dynamic population* with rolling admission and replacement of dropouts (FIGURE 12-4). For dynamic populations, the time to follow up is usually based on individual participants' dates of enrollment rather than on a fixed calendar date.

Several variants of longitudinal studies, such as time series studies and panel studies, measure the same individuals repeatedly over time, as longitudinal cohort studies do. Surveillance systems can be used to monitor whole populations over an extended period using continuous data collection rather than discrete time points. Alternatively, some types of studies measure individuals sampled from the same populations at different points in time. They do not necessarily capture the same individuals in each round of questioning. These types of studies use a series of independent cross-sectional surveys rather than a longitudinal cohort study approach.

■ 12.3 Special Considerations

For retrospective studies, the first step is to identify a source of existing records that can provide the baseline data. In some cases, existing records may also be able to provide all required follow-up data, and no contact with the individuals will be required. For retrospective studies that require contact with individuals, a method for contacting those identified in historic records will need to be developed, tested, and shown to result in a reasonable participation rate.

For a prospective study that will recruit participants based on exposure status, the first step is to identify two available sources of individuals: one for those with the exposure of interest and one for those without the exposure.

For longitudinal studies, the first step is to select a source population.

Alternatively, if the goal is to conduct secondary analysis of existing data, the first step is to identify an existing source of data. The secondary analysis of existing data is the most cost-effective way to examine study questions on two conditions:

- A completed or ongoing prospective or longitudinal cohort study has assessed the exposures and outcomes of interest.
- Electronic data files are available to outside researchers for analysis.

For prospective and longitudinal studies, decisions must be made about how often data collection will take place and how long the study (or at least the first wave of the study) will continue. Because loss of participants to follow-up before the end of the study period is a major concern of studies that follow participants forward in time, researchers must develop strategies that minimize the burden of participation and that maximize interest in continuing to participate. Some studies may increase retention rates by offering participants free medical tests or other incentives. Sufficient motivation may also be provided by reminders of the significant impact of the disease on affected persons and their family members or by notifications of the important discoveries being made as a result of their continued participation.

Once source populations have been identified, it is time to initiate data collection, as described in the next section of the book. When developing the survey instruments for cohort studies, remember the importance of establishing exposure and disease status for all participants at baseline and at follow-up. All participants must complete the same assessments to prevent the *information bias* that might result when exposed participants are more thoroughly examined for disease than unexposed participants. A strong data management system must be prepared to link baseline and follow-up data while maintaining the confidentiality of the information provided by participants. Data management is discussed in Chapter 25.

■ 12.4 Analysis: Incidence and Risk Ratios

The goal of cohort studies is to examine the incidence of new disease. The *incidence rate* is the number of new cases of disease in a population during a specified period of time divided by the total number of persons in the population who were at risk during that period. Individuals who already have the disease of interest at the start of the study period are not at risk of getting new disease, so they are removed from the denominator (FIGURE 12-5). For example, suppose a cohort study examined the incidence of disease over 1 year in a population with 50 members and that 7 of those 50 already had the disease at the start of the year. In that situation, the denominator should be

Number at risk (not diseased) at start of study period:	50 − 7 = 43	
Number of new cases:	**4**	
Incidence rate:	**4/43 = 93 per 1000**	

Number at risk (not diseased) at start of study period:	50 − 0 = 50
Number of new cases:	**15**
Incidence rate:	**15/50 = 300 per 1000**

Number at risk (not diseased) at start of study period:	50 − 25 = 25
Number of new cases:	**1**
Incidence rate:	**1/25 = 40 per 1000**

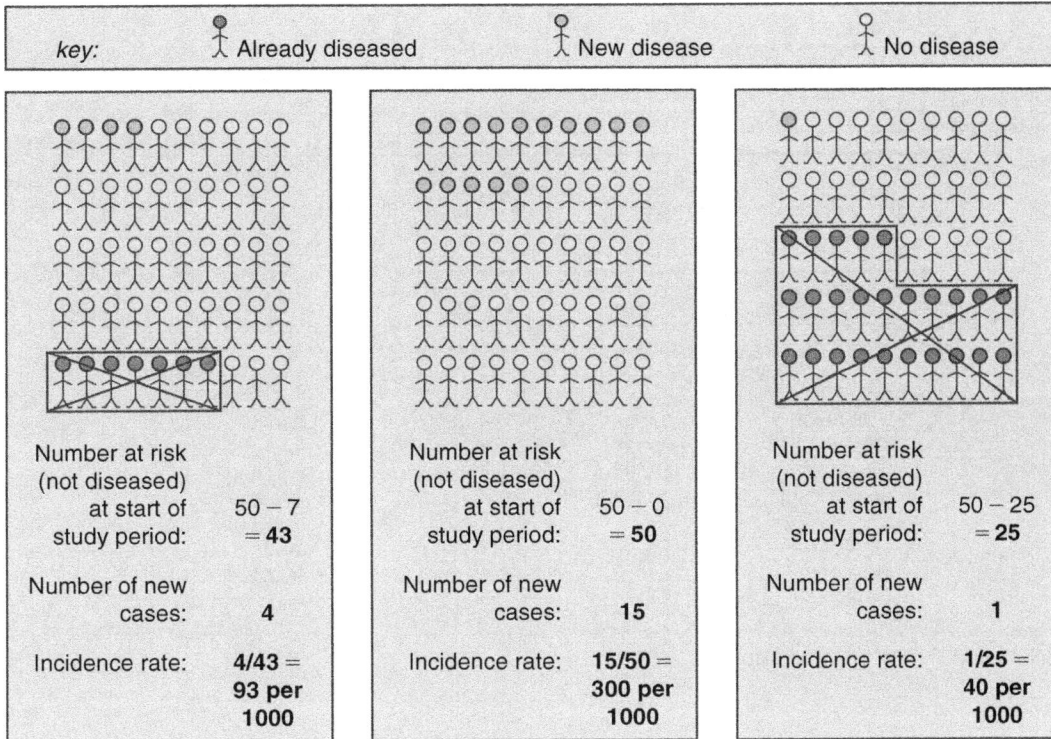

FIGURE 12-5 Incidence

43 rather than 50. If 4 of those 43 are diagnosed with the disease during the year, then the incidence rate is 4/43, or 93 per 1000 per year. (Incidence rates are often converted to units of "per 1000," "per 10,000," or the like so that they can be more easily compared.)

Some cohort studies, especially those with dynamic populations (Figure 12-4) and those that run for many years, use person-time as a denominator. *Person-time* is a way of accounting for different individuals in the study population being observed for different lengths of time. Suppose that a study recruits 10 individuals at baseline (FIGURE 12-6). After 4 years, 6 of the 10 participants are still active in the study and have not been diagnosed with the disease of interest. Together, these 6 individuals have contributed 24 person-years of observation after 4 years. Suppose that 2 of the 10 original participants are diagnosed with the disease of interest at their annual study examinations. One person is diagnosed 2 years into the study, and the other 4 years into the study. Together, these 2 individuals contributed 6 person-years of observation to the study. However, once they are diagnosed and no longer at risk of getting the disease, they are no longer able to contribute person-years to the denominator for

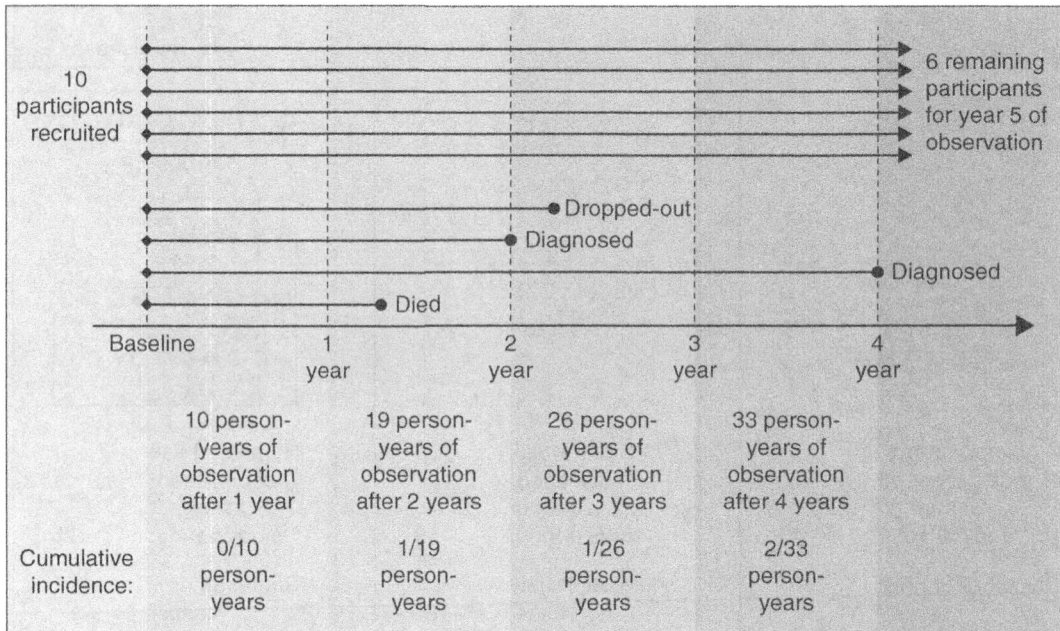

FIGURE 12-6 **Person-Year Analysis**

the calculation of incidence. Two other participants also leave the study. One drops out of the study after the second year but before the third year; this participant is considered to have contributed 2 person-years of observation. Another dies after the first year and contributes only that 1 person-year of observation. In total, over 4 years, the 10 original participants experience 2 incident cases of disease over 33 person-years of observation. For the calculation of rate ratios and other measures that rely on the comparison of incidence rates, it does not matter whether the incidence rates are measured per 1000 persons (Figure 12-5) or per 1000 person-years (Figure 12-6), as long as all incidence rates in the equation use the same units.

An initial and simple way to compare incidence rates is to compare the rates of new disease in the exposed and unexposed members of the cohort. *Excess risk*, or *attributable risk*, is the absolute difference in the incidence rate. (See FIGURE 12-7.) For example, if 10% of the unexposed and 15% of the exposed became ill during the study period, then the excess risk in the exposed was 15% – 10% = 5%. This number represents the additional risk of disease in the exposed that can be attributed to the exposure. It assumes that the exposed would have had the same rate as the unexposed if they had not had the exposure. This assumption is one of the reasons why the exposed and unexposed populations must be similar except for their exposure status.

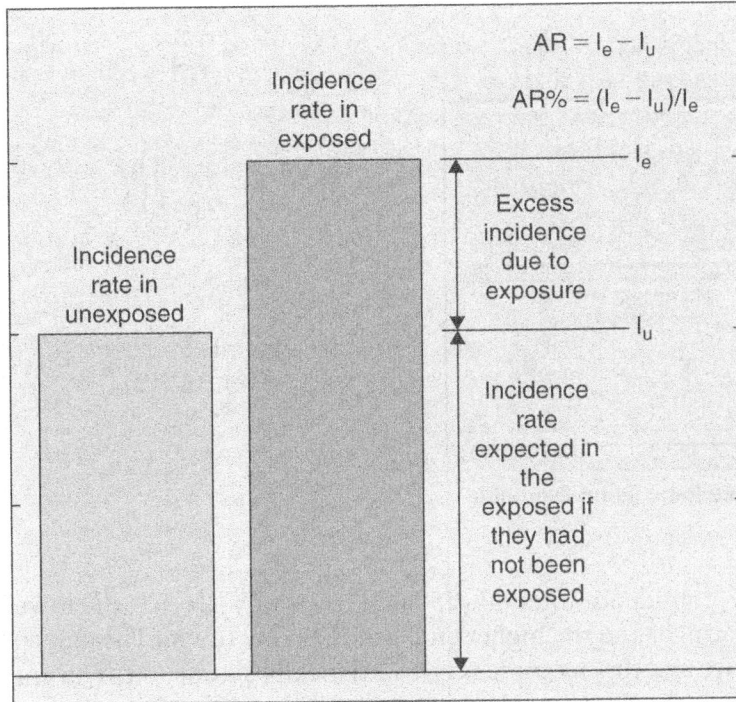

FIGURE 12-7 **Attributable (Excess) Risk**

The *attributable risk percent (AR%)* is the proportion of incident cases among the exposed that are due to the exposure. The percentage is calculated by comparing the excess risk to the incidence rate in the exposed. For the preceding example, the AR% is 5% ÷ 15% = 33%. In other words, one-third of the cases of disease in the exposed could have been prevented if the exposure was removed.

The most common measure of association for cohort studies is the *rate ratio (RR)*, also known as the *relative rate*, *risk ratio*, or *relative risk*. The RR compares the incidence rate among the exposed to the incidence rate in the unexposed (FIGURE 12-8). The RR is easy to interpret.

- If the RR is equal to 1 or close to 1, then the incidence rate was the same in the exposed and in the unexposed. The exposure is not associated with the disease.
- If the RR is greater than 1, then the incidence rate was higher in the exposed than in the unexposed. The exposure is considered risky.
- If the RR is less than 1, then the incidence rate was lower in the exposed than in the unexposed. The exposure is considered protective.

The 95% confidence interval indicates whether the RR is statistically significant (FIGURE 12-9).

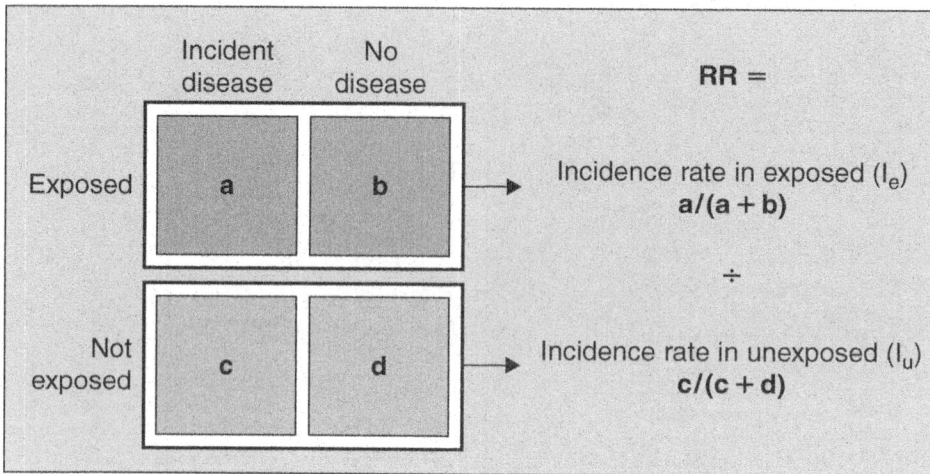

FIGURE 12-8 **Rate Ratio (Point Estimate)**

- If the 95% confidence interval (95% CI) overlaps RR = 1, the lower end is in the protective range, and the higher end is in the risky range. The association between the exposure and the outcome is not statistically significant. The appropriate conclusion is that there is no evidence for an association between the exposure and the disease.
- If the entire 95% confidence interval is less than 1, then the RR is statistically significant. The exposure is protective in the study population.
- If the entire 95% confidence interval is greater than 1, then the RR is statistically significant. The exposure is a risk factor for the disease in the study population.

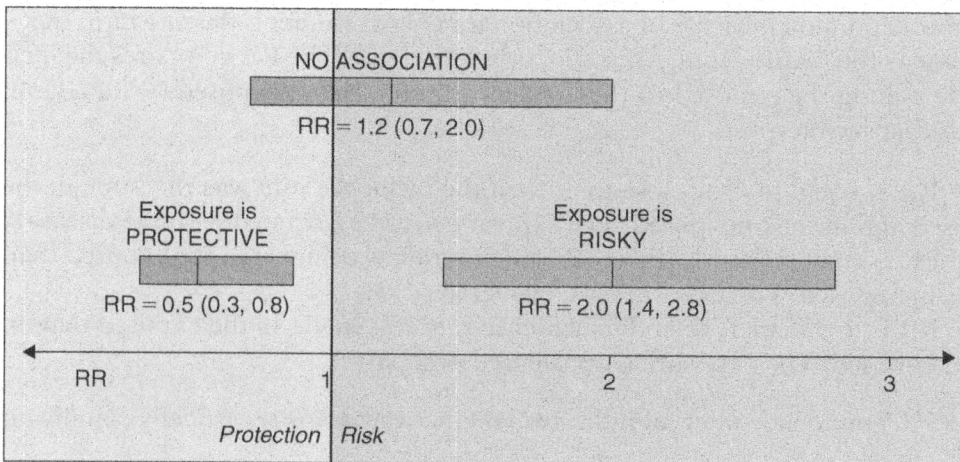

FIGURE 12-9 **Interpretation of the Rate Ratio Based on Its 95% Confidence Interval**

For the protective example in Figure 12-9, it would be accurate to report that "participants with the exposure were half as likely to develop the disease as those without the exposure." For the risky example in Figure 12-9, the report could state that "participants with the exposure were twice as likely to develop the disease as participants without the exposure."

Computer- and Internet-based statistical programs are available for the calculation of statistics that can be derived from a 2×2 table (FIGURE 12-10), such as the:

- Incidence in the exposed
- Incidence in the unexposed
- Attributable risk
- AR%

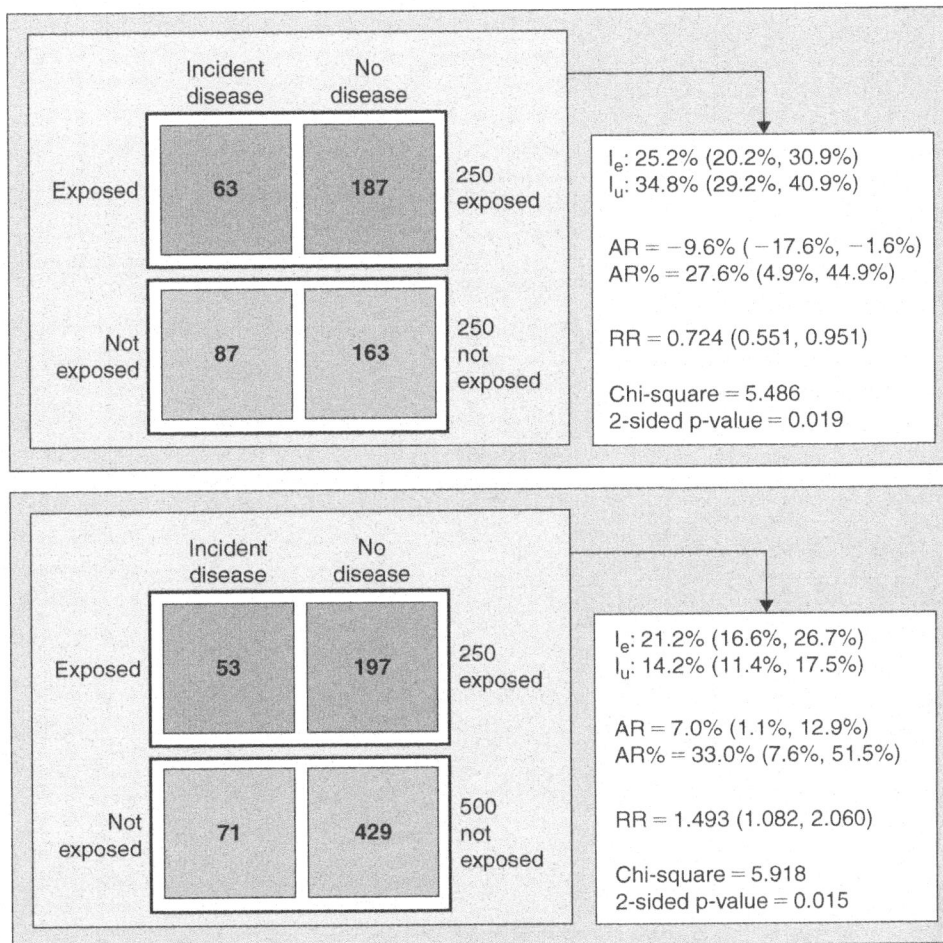

FIGURE 12-10 Examples of Rate Ratio Calculations

- RR
- 95% CI for the RR

Both examples in Figure 12-10 have statistically significant rate ratios. One example has a rate ratio of 0.724 and a 95% confidence interval of (0.551, 0.951). The exposure is considered protective because the entire 95% CI is less than 1. The other example has a rate ratio of 1.493 and a 95% confidence interval of (1.082, 2.060). The exposure is considered risky because the entire 95% CI is greater than 1.

Experimental Studies

An experimental study assigns participants to intervention and control groups in order to examine whether an intervention causes an intended outcome.

Objective	Compare outcomes in participants assigned to an intervention or control group
Primary study question	Does the exposure cause the outcome?
Population	Similar participants are randomly assigned to an intervention or control group.
When to use this approach	Assessing causality
Requirement	The experiment is ethically justifiable.
First steps	1. Decide on the intervention and eligibility criteria. 2. Define what will constitute a favorable outcome. 3. Decide what control is an appropriate comparison for the intervention. 4. Decide whether blinding will be used to prevent participants and/or the researchers who will assess outcomes from knowing whether a participant has been assigned to the intervention or the control group. 5. Select the method for randomizing participants to an intervention or control group.
What to watch out for	Noncompliance
Key statistical measure	Efficacy

FIGURE 13-1 Key Characteristics of Experimental Studies

■ 13.1 Overview

Experimental studies assign participants to receive a particular exposure (FIGURE 13-1). This is the primary distinction between an experimental study and other study designs. Observational designs (such as cross-sectional, case-control, and cohort studies) do not "do" anything to participants; they simply ask for a report on their experiences. An observational study may ask whether participants eat or do not eat an apple a day, run or do not run on a treadmill for at least 30 minutes three times each week, take or do not take a particular medicine twice a day, or have or have not seen an ad for a health promotion campaign. In contrast, an experimental study may assign some or all study participants to eat one red delicious apple daily, run on a treadmill every other day, take a pill every 12 hours, or read a health brochure.

Experimental studies are the gold standard for assessing causality. Because the researcher assigns participants to receive a particular exposure, the exact dose, duration, and frequency of the exposure are known. The researcher knows when the exposure occurred and so can compare the health status of each participant before and after the exposure. The researcher can therefore assess whether the exposure may have caused a particular outcome.

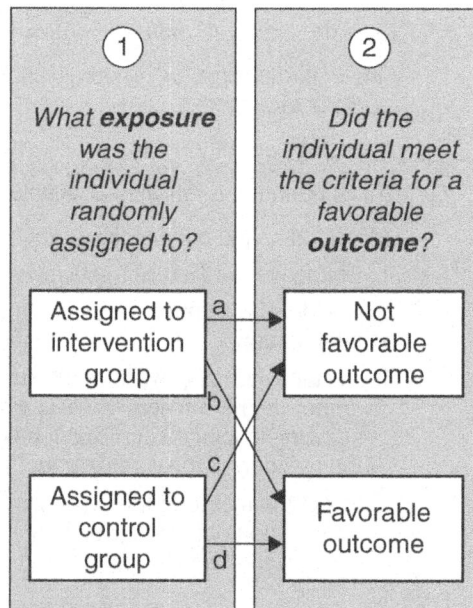

FIGURE 13-2 Framework for an Experimental Study
(The letters a, b, c, and d correspond to the equations shown in Figure 13-8.)

A typical experimental study design in the health sciences is a *randomized controlled trial (RCT)*, in which:

- Some participants are randomly assigned to an active intervention group.
- The remaining participants are assigned to a control group.
- Then all participants from both groups are followed forward in time to see who has a favorable outcome and who does not (FIGURE 13-2).

Randomized controlled trials require careful definitions of:

- The intervention
- How participants will be randomized to one of the exposure groups
- What type of control is appropriate
- What constitutes a favorable outcome for the trial

They also call for a consideration of the ethical challenges of assigning participants to an exposure, even if that exposure is expected to improve health status. These issues are discussed in the following sections.

13.2 Describing the Intervention

The first step in an experimental study is to carefully define the intervention that participants assigned to the active intervention group will receive. The description should state exactly:

- What the intervention will be
- Where and how participants will receive the intervention
- When, how often, and for what duration participants will receive the intervention
- The eligibility criteria for participants

For example, a new drug trial will declare very strict requirements for the composition of the pill to be ingested, how often it will be taken, for how many weeks it will be taken, and who will meet the case definition for eligibility to participate. A new strength-building intervention will provide detailed descriptions of the exercise procedures and how they will change in intensity over the study period, how participants will be coached or supervised, where participants will engage in the exercises, how long the study period will last, and what inclusion and exclusion criteria will apply to potential volunteers.

13.3 Defining Outcomes

Most experimental studies are superiority trials that aim to demonstrate that a new intervention is better than some type of control (FIGURE 13-3). Some studies aim instead

Goal	Success
Superiority trial	The intervention is better than the control.
Noninferiority trial	The intervention is not worse than the control.
Equivalence trial	The intervention is equal to the control.

FIGURE 13-3 Types of Success

Intervention	Intended Outcome	Favorable Outcome for an Individual	Unfavorable Outcome for an Individual	Favorable Outcome for the Study Population
New diet- and exercise-based weight-loss program	Significant weight loss	The loss of ≥10% body weight and maintenance of lower weight for ≥6 months	The loss of <10% body weight or failure to maintain weight loss of ≥10% or more for ≥6 months	The proportion of those who lose at least 10% of their body weight and maintain that loss for at least 6 months is higher in the intervention group than in the control group.
New drug therapy	Improvement of the quality of life for those with a particular disease condition	Improvement in quality of life	Failure to demonstrate improvement in quality of life	The rate of improvement in the drug therapy (intervention) group is higher than the improvement rate in the placebo (control) group, according to a carefully defined and validated set of criteria for what constitutes improvement.
New preventive vaccine	The prevention of infection	Incident infection does not occur.	Incident infection occurs.	The incidence of infection in the vaccinated (intervention) group is lower than the incidence of infection in the unvaccinated (control) group, as confirmed by laboratory testing.

FIGURE 13-4 Examples of Favorable Outcomes

to show that the new treatment is as good or no worse than existing interventions. "Better" could mean that an intervention is better than a current therapy at curing existing disease, or it could mean that a new intervention is better than a placebo at preventing new disease from occurring. Because the term "better" can be defined in so many ways, the researcher must carefully define what constitutes a favorable outcome for the experiment. Because the data collected during the study are intended to show whether a better outcome was achieved, the measure of success must be stipulated prior to the initiation of the study.

For example, an individual participant's success in a weight-loss program could be defined as the loss of at least 10% body weight and the maintenance of the lower weight for at least 6 months (FIGURE 13-4). Alternatively, success could be defined as the loss of at least 15 pounds over a 2-month intervention period or as achieving a body mass index (BMI) of less than 30 by the end of the study period.

If the goal of a study is to test whether a new drug is better than a placebo at improving the quality of life of those with a particular disease condition, the definition of "improved quality of life" should be carefully considered and validated. This can be done by means of clinical examinations and/or survey instruments designed to assess various aspects of quality of life. If the goal is to evaluate whether a new vaccine prevents infection, then laboratory tests should be used to confirm the presence or absence of past, recent, and/or current infection.

■ 13.4 Selecting Controls

Experimental studies usually assign some participants to the active intervention and the remainder to a control group (FIGURE 13-5). The most typical control is a *placebo*, an inactive comparison that is similar to the therapy being tested. Examples of placebos are a sugar pill used as a control for a pill with an active medication, a saline injection used as a control for an injection of an active substance, and a sham procedure that is designed to look and feel like a real clinical procedure used as a control for that active procedure.

The mere act of taking a pill or receiving some other form of therapy, even if it is inert or inactive, is often enough to make recipients feel better and/or behave better. Placebo-controlled studies allow the effect of the active therapy to be examined separately from the boost in health status that people may experience simply by participating in a research project or receiving some sort of intervention.

It is sometimes unethical to use a placebo when an effective therapy is already available. However, if the goal of the experiment is to see whether a new therapy is better than a current one, then it is appropriate to compare the new therapy to some existing "standard of care," whether that is the best therapy currently available or the standard local therapy. Sometimes the new therapy may be given in addition to the existing therapy.

Type of Control	Active Intervention	Comparison
Placebo/inactive comparison	Active pill	Inactive pill
	Injection of an active substance	Injection of saline solution
	Acupuncture needles inserted at acupuncture points	Acupuncture needles inserted at locations in the body that are not acupuncture points (sham acupuncture)
	Some other active ingredient	An inactive substance that is indistinguishable from the active intervention in terms of appearance, odor, taste, texture, and delivery mechanism
Active comparison/ standard of care	New therapy	Current best therapy for the condition being studied
	New therapy	Current standard therapy
	New therapy	Some other existing therapy
	Current therapy plus new therapy	Current therapy alone
Dose-response	Some dose of a medication	Alternate doses of the medication
	Some duration of a therapy	Alternate durations of the therapy
No intervention	New intervention	Participants assigned to the control group are asked to maintain their normal routines.
Self	New intervention	Each participant's status before the intervention is compared to his or her own status after the intervention.
	New intervention	Each participant receives the new intervention for some duration and the comparison for some duration, preferably in a random order.

FIGURE 13-5 Examples of Types of Controls

Sometimes the goal is to determine how much of an intervention is required. For example, should the dose of a substance be changed? (Is 100 mg of a medication as effective as 200 mg?) Or should the duration of therapy be reconsidered? (Do 4 weeks of physical therapy work as well as 8 weeks?) In such cases, varying doses and durations may be tested and compared to one another. Sometimes different interventions are compared in various combinations in one study using a factorial study design.

Although experimental studies sometimes involve a control group of participants who are randomly assigned to maintain their normal routines, this method is usually not preferred. The approach raises ethical concerns about discouraging the adoption of healthier lifestyles during the course of the study. It also raises concerns about a type of bias called the *Hawthorne effect* that can occur when participants in a study change their behavior for the better. For example, suppose a researcher is initiating a study of a new weight-loss program and plans to randomly assign participants either to the new therapy or to a normal routine group. In this situation, simply informing the controls that they will be weighed at the start and end of the study period will be enough to spur a sizable proportion of the control group to initiate an exercise program, start eating a healthier diet, or take other steps to lose weight. These changes may interfere with the accurate measurement of the impact of the new intervention.

When there are ethical concerns about the appropriateness of assigning some participants to a potentially risky intervention or about not assigning all participants to a potentially life-saving intervention, sometimes participants can serve as their own controls. Sometimes each participant's status before the intervention is compared to his or her own status after the intervention. The results of this experimental design are not as clear-cut as using a placebo because time alone can lead to significant improvements or declines in health status, especially among those who are severely ill. When possible, it is advisable to use what is called a *crossover design*. In this approach, the researcher assigns some participants first to the active intervention and then the control and assigns other participants first to the control and then to the active intervention.

◼ 13.5 Blinding

Blinding, sometimes called *masking*, occurs when participants in an experimental study and perhaps some research team members do not know whether a participant is in the active intervention group or the control group. In a *single-blind study*, participants are unaware of their exposure status. In a *double-blind study*, neither the participants nor the persons assessing the participants' health status know which participants are in the active and control groups.

Blinding minimizes the information bias that can occur if participants or assessors are able to assess outcomes differently based on the results they expect for an exposure. For example, blinding prevents participants in the active intervention group from reporting more favorable results because they expect a positive outcome. Blinding also prevents assessors from recording more favorable results, either intentionally or unintentionally, for participants in the active intervention group.

Blinding is usually possible only when all participants are assigned to similar exposures. If participants in both the active intervention group and the control group are taking pills (of the same color, shape, size, and taste), if both are getting injections, or if both are participating in similar exercise programs, a blinded study may be possible. In contrast, if the active intervention is a special diet and the controls eat their usual diets, if the active group will participate in exercise classes and the controls will be on their own, or if the active intervention will include both diet and exercise components and the control only a diet plan, then a blinded study may not be possible. To minimize the likelihood of bias in studies that are not blinded, it is helpful to identify objective outcome measures (such as laboratory tests) rather than subjective outcome measures (such as participants' self-reported feelings).

■ 13.6 Randomizing

A variety of approaches can be used to randomly allocate participants to an active intervention group or a control group (FIGURE 13-6).

- *Simple randomization* uses a coin toss, a random number generator, or some other simple mechanism to assign each individual to one of the groups.
- *Block randomization* randomly assigns groups of people, such as whole communities or whole schools, to an intervention or control group.

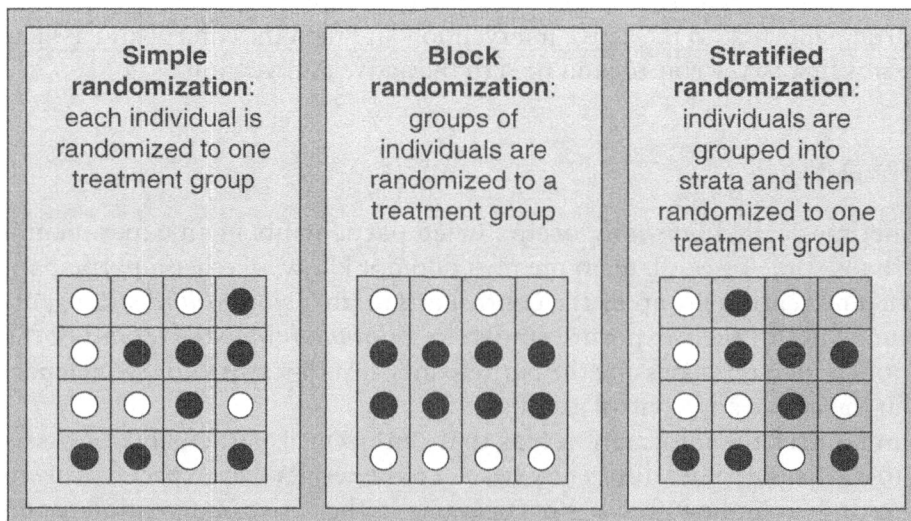

FIGURE 13-6 Examples of Types of Randomization

- *Stratified randomization* randomly assigns individuals within certain subgroups (such as males and females or various age groups) to a particular exposure. This type of randomization is useful when simple randomization may not result in enough members of certain subgroups being randomized to each of the exposure groups.

Reference books that focus specifically on experimental studies provide additional details about methods for randomization.

■ 13.7 Ethical Considerations

All research with human participants or their personal data raises ethical concerns that researchers must address, but experimental studies involve a particularly high level of ethical risk. In experimental studies, the researcher assigns participants to exposures that the participants do not choose and may have been unlikely to encounter in normal life had they not volunteered to participate in a research project. This means that a number of issues must be considered before initiating an experimental study (FIGURE 13-7). For example:

- The principle of *equipoise* states that experimental research should be conducted only when there is genuine uncertainty about which treatment will work better.
- The principle of *distributive justice* implies that the source population must be an appropriate one and that the research must not exploit low-resource individuals who are unlikely to have continued access to the therapy if it is found to be successful.
- The principle of *respect for persons* requires two things of participants: (1) that they volunteer for a study without being unduly influenced by the prospect of being compensated for their participation and (2) that they are able to understand what it means to be a research subject, including the possibility of being assigned to a control group instead of the new intervention.

Study topic	Recruitment	Randomization	Data collection	Follow-up
Is the study really necessary? (equipoise)	Is the source population an appropriate and justifiable one?	Do participants truly understand that they may not receive the active intervention?	How will adverse outcomes be monitored and addressed?	What happens if a participant experiences study-related harm after the conclusion of the study?
Is an experimental design truly necessary?	Is the inducement to participate appropriate?	Is it appropriate to use a placebo? Is it appropriate to use some other control?	When might an experiment need to be discontinued early?	Will participants have continuing access to the therapy if it is shown to be successful?

FIGURE 13-7 Examples of Ethical Issues to Consider When Planning an Experimental Study

- The principles of *beneficence* and *nonmaleficence* require that researchers balance the likely benefits and risks of the study. For example, researchers must consider the use of a placebo or another control, put in place a monitoring system for adverse reactions, and identify the conditions under which an experiment would be discontinued early. The study could be discontinued either because one of the exposures proves to be risky or because the new intervention appears to be so beneficial that keeping it from the control group would be unethical.

Chapter 21 discusses additional ethical principles that must be considered when planning and conducting research with human subjects. Research ethics committee review is required for all experimental studies, as explained in Chapter 22.

■ 13.8 Analysis

Experimental studies use many of the same measures of association that cohort studies do, including relative rates, attributable risks (excess risk or risk reduction), attributable risk percentages, and measures of survival. Cohort studies use these measures to examine the impact of an unassigned exposure on the incidence of disease. Experimental studies use them to examine the impact of an assigned exposure on the likelihood of having either a favorable or unfavorable outcome.

Also, several measures are specific to experimental studies.

- *Efficacy* is the proportion of individuals in the control group who experience an unfavorable outcome who could have been expected to have a favorable outcome had they been in the active group instead (FIGURE 13-8). A high efficacy is an indicator that an intervention is successful.
- The *number needed to treat (NNT)* is the expected number of people who would have to receive a treatment to prevent an unfavorable outcome in one person (or, alternately stated, to achieve a favorable outcome in one person). A small NNT indicates a more effective intervention. If a drug is intended to prevent stroke and has an NNT of 5, then 5 people have to take the drug for one year (or some other specified time period) to prevent one of the 5 from having a stroke. If the drug has an NNT of 102, it means that 102 people have to take the drug to prevent one of the 102 from having a stroke.
- A related concept is the *number needed to harm (NNH)*, which is the number of people who would need to receive a particular treatment in order to expect that one of them would have a particular adverse outcome. A large NNH indicates a more effective intervention. NNT and NNH are often used for cost-effectiveness analysis.

Another special consideration is whether to use a *treatment-received approach*, which limits analysis to the participants who were fully compliant with their assigned intervention.

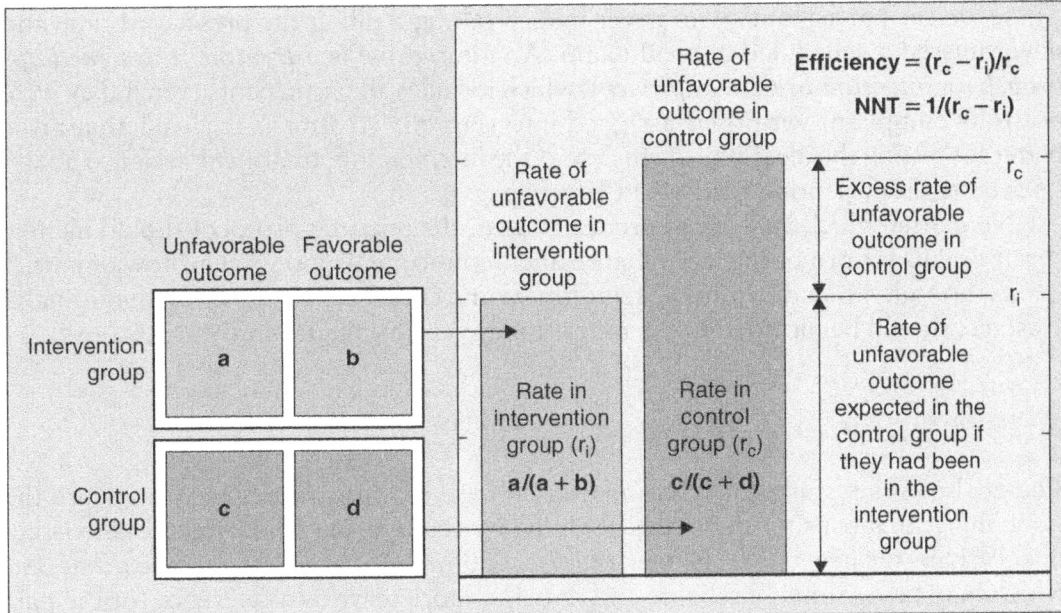

FIGURE 13-8 Efficacy and Number Needed to Treat (NNT)

Efficiency $= (r_c - r_i)/r_c$

NNT $= 1/(r_c - r_i)$

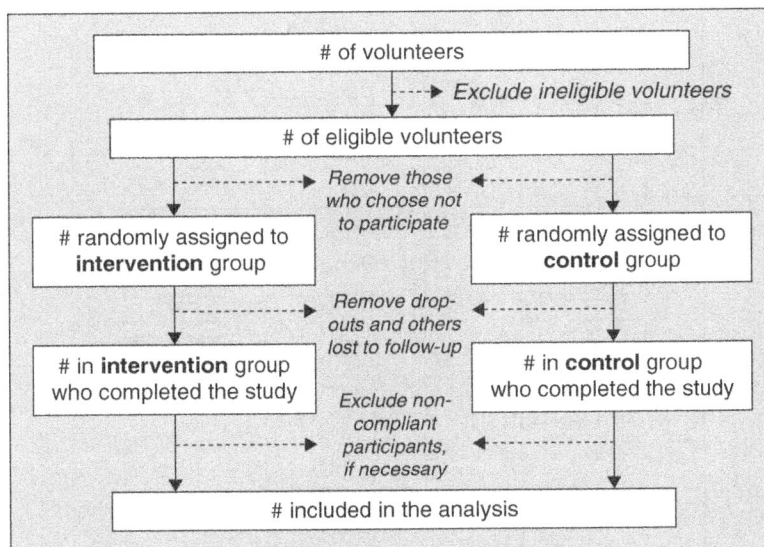

FIGURE 13-9 Flow of Participants in an Experimental Study

These are the participants who never missed taking a pill at the prescribed time and never missed a scheduled clinical exam. An alternative is a *treatment-assigned approach* (or *intention-to-treat approach*), which includes all participants even if they were not fully compliant with their assigned intervention. Treatment-received analysis is better for testing the ideal-world efficacy of the intervention; treatment-assigned analysis is better at measuring real-world effectiveness.

No matter which analytic approach is used, the research protocol should include specific plans for promoting compliance and minimizing dropouts. The flow of participants through the study, from the recruitment and enrollment stage through the analysis stage, should be included in the report for any experimental study (FIGURE 13-9).

■ 13.9 Screening and Diagnostic Tests

The goal of some studies is to compare two tests that are supposed to measure the same thing. In most situations, this goal involves comparing a new test to an existing one. Perhaps the new test is cheaper, quicker, and/or less invasive than the current test, which may be reasonably reliable and may therefore serve as a reference for the participant's "actual" status. For example, a new blood antigen test for a type of cancer may be compared to biopsy results. Most trials of laboratory-based tests can be considered observational because they do not require the researchers to do anything to the

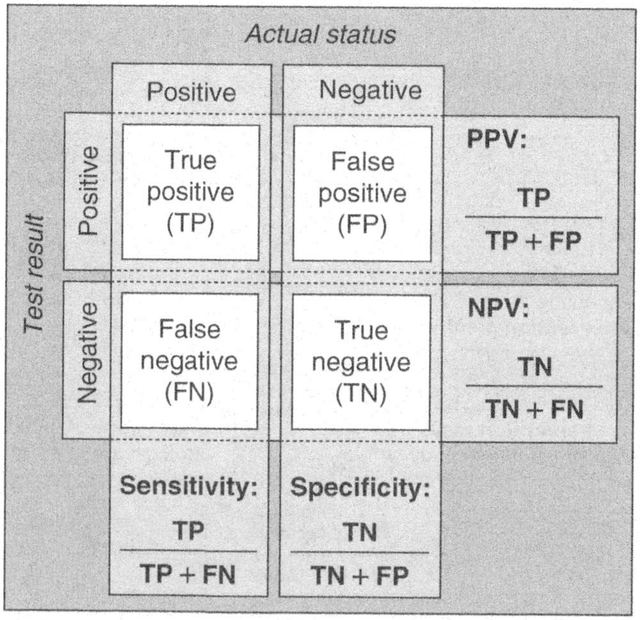

FIGURE 13-10 **Test Results**

participants other than collect a biological specimen. Other tests involve experimental procedures and are appropriately classified as experimental.

Studies of new screening and diagnostic tests should have a clear set of eligibility criteria. They may call for intentionally seeking out some individuals known to have the disease of interest and some known to be disease free. An appropriate reference standard must be identified, and a rationale for any cutoff points for the new test and reference test should be determined. For example, the protocol should specify the concentration of antigens in the blood that will indicate a positive versus a negative test result. A system should be put in place to ensure that the examiners—the clinicians or laboratory scientists conducting the assessments—are blinded to the "actual" status of the participants as indicated by the reference test.

FIGURE 13-10 shows how to calculate the sensitivity, specificity, positive predictive value, and negative predictive value of new screening or diagnostic tests in comparison to a reference standard. The *sensitivity* is the proportion of people who actually have a disease (according to the reference standard) who test positive (using the new test). The *specificity* is the proportion of people who do not have the disease who test negative. The *positive predictive value (PPV)* is the proportion of those who test positive who actually have the disease. The *negative predicitive value (NPV)* is the proportion of those who test negative who actually do not have the disease. A good screening or diagnostic test will have high values for each of these measures.

Similar statistics can be used to determine the extent of agreement between two assessors who are evaluating the same study participants. For example, a measurement known as the *kappa statistic* can indicate whether two radiologists examining the same set of X-rays reach the same conclusion about the presence or absence of a fracture more or less often than expected by chance. Other measurements of *inter-observer agreement* (also called *concordance*) can also be used to assess the validity and consistency of assessment tools and procedures. More detailed information about quality-control techniques is available in a variety of reference books.

Qualitative Studies

A qualitative study looks for the themes and meanings that emerge from the observation and evaluation of a situation or context.

■ 14.1 Qualitative Study Methods

Qualitative data collection is not a detached, structured process based on a random sample of individuals. Instead, researchers have intense contact with a selected group of informants (often identified by means of purposive sampling). The researchers are allowed to express empathy and, when appropriate, to be *participant observers*, who gain access to and understanding of a community by immersing in its practices. Because qualitative researchers are so closely engaged with participants, they need to reflect on how their backgrounds might bias their observations, and they need to be transparent about these potential limitations when reporting findings.

A carefully considered approach is used to gather and interpret data. For example:

- *Phenomenology* seeks to understand how participants understand, interpret, and find meaning in their own unique life experiences and feelings.
- *Grounded theory* is an inductive reasoning process that uses observations to develop general theories that explain human behavior.

- *Ethnography* aims to develop an insider's view (an *emic perspective*), rather than an outsider's view (an *etic perspective*), of how members of a particular cultural group see their world.

A set of somewhat flexible techniques is used to ensure the comprehensiveness of the collected information. This approach may involve a combination of listening and watching, with field notes being taken to record both verbal and nonverbal cues.

Two of the most common methods used to collect data are in-depth interviews and focus groups.

- *In-depth* and *semi-structured interviews* of individuals use open-ended questions to explore viewpoints. The interviewer is allowed to probe for more details about any response in order to gain fuller understanding of the participant's experiences and perspectives.
- *Focus groups* of about 4 to 12 people are moderated discussions led by a facilitator from the research team. The facilitator encourages participants to interact with one another and to clarify their individual and shared perspectives.

Interviews and focus groups are usually audio- or video-recorded, then transcribed so that the exact words (and sometimes also the nonverbal expressions) can be coded and interpreted. Interviews are often supplemented by other methods, such as participant diaries or journals. The analysis of qualitative data usually involves coding and classifying observations (sometimes using software designed for this purpose) and deriving major and minor themes from the groups of observations. Reports of the findings of qualitative studies often incorporate quotations that express participants' perspectives and experiences in their own words.

Qualitative research can stand alone, or it can be used in conjunction with quantitative studies. Before initiating any qualitative study, researchers should consult specialty references or experts in qualitative methods.

■ 14.2 Consensus Methods

The goal of some studies is to identify areas of consensus and areas of contention among individuals who are experts on a particular topic and/or a particular community or organization. The results of the deliberations are then used, for example, to select research priorities, to identify best practices, and to agree on plans of action.

Several techniques have been developed for shaping these conversations and the resulting conclusions. For example, the *Delphi method* is a structured decision-making and forecasting process in which participants engage in several rounds of:

- Completing individual questionnaires
- A facilitator summarizing and sharing the responses

- Panelists reconsidering their perspectives after reflecting on the opinic
  by others

The goal is for each iteration to move the panel of experts closer to agree.

■ 14.3 Program Evaluation

Program evaluation includes a variety of approaches for examining the goals, processes, and/or outcomes of projects (specific, time-limited activities), programs (ongoing groups of projects), and/or policies. The goal of these assessments is usually not to identify what is being done correctly or incorrectly, but to provide feedback about what is working well and what can and should be improved.

In the health sciences, a typical evaluation begins with a meeting at which stakeholders describe the purposes of the program, how it was intended to function, how it is actually functioning, and what they themselves hope to learn from the assessment. Based on these conversations, an evaluation approach is selected. Evidence is gathered from a variety of sources, possibly including a review of existing program documents, surveys of stakeholders, interviews with key informants, and observations at program sites. All the evidence is then reviewed and categorized, perhaps using a framework like SWOT. *SWOT* identifies *s*trengths (internal organizational strengths), *w*eaknesses (internal organizational limitations), *o*pportunities (external strengths), and *t*hreats (external limitations, which might be political, economic, sociocultural, technological, environmental, or legal). Finally, practical suggestions are made based on the conclusions of the assessment.

A similar process can be used as a component of other forms of evaluative research, such as:

- Needs assessment
- Cost-effectiveness analysis
- Health services research, which examines factors related to the types of health services and providers available to a population, the organization and financing of those health services, and the impact of governments and policies on population health

Designing the Study and Collecting Data

Identify study question	Select study approach	Design study & collect data	Analyze data	Report findings

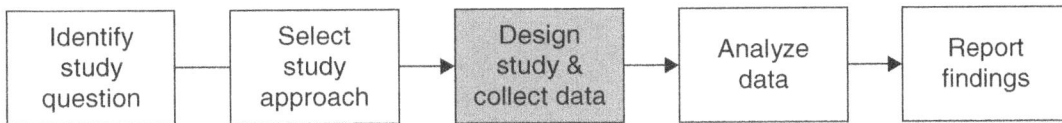

The third step in the research process is to develop and implement a detailed study plan. This section describes how to create a protocol for primary, secondary, and tertiary studies.

- Overview: developing a proposal and protocol
- Primary studies: collecting new data
  - Selecting a sample population
  - Estimating sample size
  - Developing a questionnaire
  - Surveys and interviews
  - Additional assessments
  - Ethical considerations
  - Ethical review and approval
- Secondary studies: existing data sets
- Tertiary studies: systematic reviews and meta-analyses

Overview: Developing a Proposal and Protocol

A proposal is usually a request for funding or for supervisory approval. A protocol is a detailed handbook describing all the actions that will be taken during the implementation of the study.

■ 15.1 Overview of Research Plans by Study Approach

Once a study question and a study approach have been selected, the next step is to create a detailed research plan. The components of this plan will vary somewhat according to the study approach (FIGURE 15-1). For the collection of new data from individuals, the researcher needs to:

- Develop a questionnaire and other data collection tools
- Identify an appropriate way to recruit participants
- Select methods for collecting and recording responses from participants
- Prepare an application for a research ethics review committee

If existing data will be analyzed, an appropriate data file must be identified and the data set and supporting materials acquired. If a literature review will be conducted, the search strategy must be defined, eligible articles identified, and relevant information from each article extracted into a database. For all study plans, it is helpful to create a protocol that will guide each step of the data collection and management process.

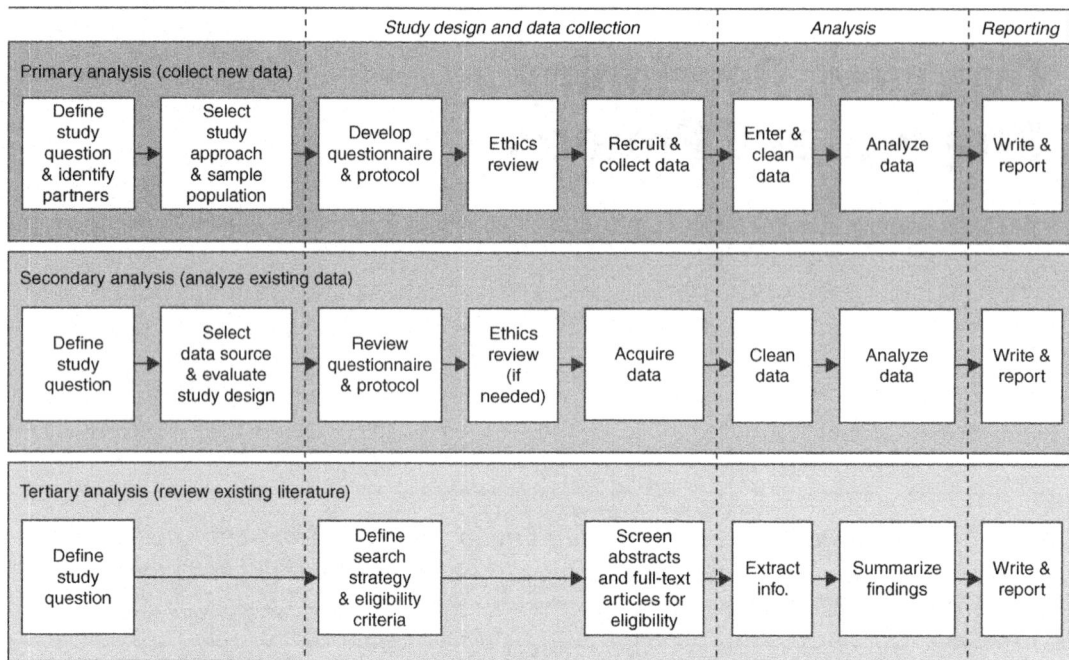

FIGURE 15-1 Research Plans for Primary, Secondary, and Tertiary Data Collection

■ 15.2 Resources for Research

A first step in creating a research plan is to assess all the resources available for the research project and all the resources that are expected to be required. The aim is to ensure that the anticipated resources are adequate for the intended study design. Many research projects require little in the way of material resources. A secondary analysis or review article may require only access to a computer, a statistical software program, and a decent collection of electronic journals. Some primary studies incur only relatively minor expenses, such as the cost of photocopying a limited number of questionnaires. Other primary studies may become quite expensive. They may, for example, involve travel to a distant field site, laboratory testing or other clinical assessments, lengthy durations of data collection, and/or the hiring of interviewers and data entry personnel.

Money and materials are not the only resources to consider. For many studies, the most important resources are the individuals who are available to contribute their time, expertise, and/or connections to the project. (See Chapter 5 for information about working with collaborators.) Other resources may include things like access to:

- Potential study participants or data sets (perhaps through a personal contact, a professional organization, a community organization, or a patient or client database)

- Laboratory space, office space, or a meeting room
- Equipment, such as computers and copying machines

■ 15.3 Funding Sources and Budgets

Although not all research projects require financial support, sometimes projects need outside sources of money, or, at a minimum, they would be significantly enhanced by them. Common sources of funding are *internal grants* from a school or employer and *external grants* from private foundations, corporations, government agencies, or other sources.

A proposal must align with the goals of the sponsoring agency and its typical funding level. Some organizations support only research focused on a very specific disease or population, and others are much more general in scope. Some student-focused awards consist of only a few hundred dollars, and some government agencies distribute millions of dollars to established researchers.

Granting agencies prefer to fund research projects that will answer well-defined and significant study questions and that have a budget appropriate for the work to be done. The budget should cover all the essential costs of the research project without being excessive in its total amount or in any category. A student or trainee applying for a small grant may want to request funding for only basic direct expenses, such as travel and photocopying. A larger grant may request:

- Salary support for core members of the research team
- Stipends for consultants
- Funds for the purchase of equipment and supplies
- Funds for administrative costs (such as payments for facilities usage, utilities, communications, and support staff)
- Funds for compensating or reimbursing the expenses of study participants

It is not unusual for the funding cap from a source such as a competitive student research award to be lower than the actual amount required for a project. In this situation, the researcher should show in the grant application which expenses will be paid by the new grant, if funded, and which will be covered by other sources. When submitting a proposal, the researcher should also ascertain the absolute minimum amount of support required and, if adequate funds cannot be secured, be prepared to abandon a project (and forgo possible offers of financial support for that specific project). For example, if transportation and photocopying costs will be $800 and funding is secured for only $250, the researcher may decide to use the time, energy, and money elsewhere.

Funding rates are often extremely low, and processing time varies. Waiting for funding can stall projects for lengthy periods of time.

■ 15.4 Research Timelines and Responsibilities

Most research proposals and protocols include a fairly detailed schedule for the planned research project. It is therefore helpful to:

- Create a list of all the steps from planning the study through the dissemination of results
- Create a calendar that shows when each of these steps is expected to begin and end
- Set deadlines along the way that will help ensure that the project stays on track toward timely completion

The schedule will need to be somewhat flexible because predicting how long some steps will take can be difficult. For example, waiting for ethics approval or for the disbursement of funds from a granting agency might take several months instead of several weeks. Data collection might be completed far more slowly (or more quickly) than expected. Data entry might take much more time than originally anticipated. Additionally, relying on collaborators to complete some aspects of the work may result in delays. This is especially likely when the lead researcher is not in a position of authority. For example, a student researcher might not be able to push for a faster response when a supervisor is slow to provide feedback. Sometimes these holdups are not a major concern. However, missed deadlines may be a serious problem when some collaborators have inflexible schedules or are completing degree requirements.

Research projects proceed most smoothly when all research team members have the same understanding about each person's roles and responsibilities. The protocol should include dates for the completion of all tasks and the incentives or reminders to be used to encourage careful and on-time completion. It may also be helpful to identify a process for resolving conflicts. Sometimes one person, often a senior researcher, is designated to adjudicate delays in the submissions of agreed-upon deliverables, disagreements about the interpretation of the protocol or the nature of an assigned task, and other differences of opinion or awkward situations.

Universities, hospitals, and other institutions typically require one researcher to act as the *primary investigator* (PI) and to accept responsibility for guaranteeing that:

- The protocol is followed.
- Any adverse outcomes are immediately reported to the institution's research ethics committee.
- The budget is properly managed.

In some situations the PI is the person doing the greatest amount of work on the project, but many institutions require a senior employee to be designated as the PI. For example, some universities require a professor to be listed as the primary investigator on any research project that involves human subjects, even if a student is taking the lead role in the conduct of the project.

Background

- Brief summary of what is already known about the topic
  - Literature review, with citations of the previous work of other researchers
  - Summary of the researcher's own previous work on the topic and any preliminary results (if applicable)
- Purpose of the new project
- Significance and importance of the new project
- Definition of key terms

Goals and specific measurable or testable aims, objectives, or hypotheses

Methods and procedures

- Study design
- Source population (for new data collection) or data source (for analysis of existing data)
- Sampling methodology and expected sample size
- Recruiting procedures (for new data collection)
- Definition and measurement of key variables
- Data collection procedures
- Laboratory procedures (if applicable)

Analysis plan

- Data management plan
- Data analysis plan

Dissemination plan

References

Timeline

Budget and justification (Not all items will be applicable to all projects.)

- Personnel (salaries and benefits)
- Equipment and supplies for the office (such as computers, software programs, printers and photocopiers, and paper) and laboratory (if applicable)
- Communications (such as postage, phones, and Internet access)
- Travel (including mileage on cars, parking, local transportation, and possibly airfare, hotels, and food)
- Other costs (such as publication fees and overhead costs paid to the institution by some funding agencies)

Researcher information (such as a biosketch, CV, or résumé)

Optional appendices

- Questionnaire or other survey instrument
- Research ethics review application and supporting documents

FIGURE 15-2 Typical Proposal Content

◼ 15.5 Writing a Research Proposal

Most granting agencies require the submission of a formal research proposal, and students and employees conducting research are often expected to submit a proposal for review by supervisors. Most research proposals (FIGURE 15-2) contain:

- A brief background that explains the importance of the proposed project
- A goals statement
- A description of the methods that will be used
- An analysis plan
- A plan for the dissemination of findings
- A timeline
- A budget
- Basic information about the researchers

The application guidelines usually provide specifications about what content should be included in a proposal, how the proposal should be organized, and how long each section should be.

◼ 15.6 Writing a Research Protocol

The research proposal serves as the backbone for developing a very detailed research protocol. The protocol explains the exact procedures that will be used for every step of the research process. For a primary study, the protocol will explain, among other things:

- The exact processes that will be used for contacting and recruiting participants.
- The desired sample size and the steps that will be taken to acquire an adequate number of participants.
- The exact procedures that will be used to obtain and document informed consent (or to document refusal to participate).
- The exact questions that will be asked (and, if interviews will be used to gather information from participants, the exact instructions for how those questions will be asked).
- The exact codes for the entry of various responses to survey questions (including missing responses) into the computer database.
- The exact steps that will be taken to maintain the confidentiality of any personal information that might be contained in that data set.
- If applicable, the research protocol must also describe in detail any laboratory procedure that might be used.

For a systematic review, the protocol is quite different but equally detailed. It defines the exact criteria for an article's eligibility for inclusion in the review. It spells out exactly how articles that cannot easily be classified according to the eligibility criteria will be handled. For all study designs, the protocol should anticipate likely dilemmas and areas of confusion and address them as completely as possible.

Ideally, a protocol should:

- Fully describe all the procedures that will be used for data collection and analysis.
- Provide details about the responsibilities of each member of the research team.
- List the deadlines for completion of all the steps in the research process.
- Describe the mechanism for updating any part of the research plan, should the need arise after approval of the initial protocol. (Significant adjustments to the protocol may need to be approved by all relevant research ethics committees before they can be implemented.)

A strong protocol provides enough detail that another researcher could easily replicate the study. It should also be detailed enough that the entire methods section of any paper that will result from the project could be written before data collection begins.

■ 15.7 Preparing for Data Collection

Before initiating data collection, make sure that all preparations have been finalized.

- Are all supplies and equipment ready for use?
- Have all collaborators approved of their designated roles, responsibilities, and deadlines?
- Have all collaborators completed any required ethics training?
- Have the final versions of all study documents (such as the informed consent statement and the questionnaire) been approved by all relevant research ethics committees, if required?
- Has the data management system been tested and found to be reliable?
- If applicable, are all participating laboratories ready to begin processing samples?

The following chapters provide information about some of the essential steps in preparing for primary data collection: identifying a sample population, developing a questionnaire and other forms of assessment, and ensuring that ethical standards are followed.

Primary Studies: Selecting a Sample Population

A source of study participants for primary studies should be identified early in the research process.

16.1 Types of Research Populations

At least four different types of populations must be considered when preparing to collect data (FIGURE 16-1). (Several different names are used to describe these four entities, but the concepts are the same for all health science fields.)

- The broadest group is the *target population* to which the results of the study should be applicable.
- The *source population* is a well-defined subset of individuals from the target population.
- The *sample population* consists of the individuals from the source population who are asked to participate.
- The *study population* consists of the eligible members of the sample population who consent to participate in the study.

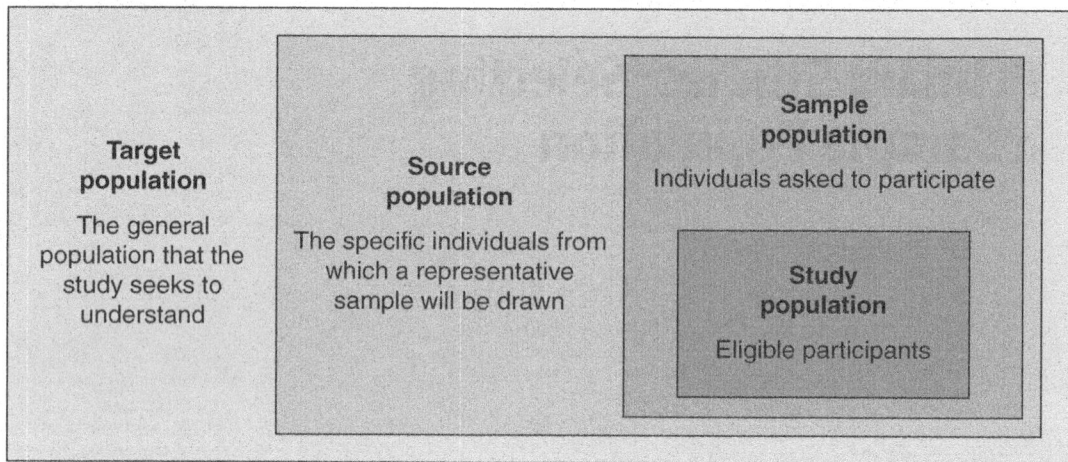

FIGURE 16-1 The Study Population Is a Subset of Individuals Sampled from a Source Population

■ 16.2 Target and Source Populations

A well-defined study question identifies a target population to which the results of the study should apply. A target population might be quite narrow. The goal might be to identify the cause of an outbreak of a drug-resistant bacterial strain in one wing of a long-term acute care hospital. Or the goal might be to measure the prevalence of binge drinking on one college campus. Alternatively, the target population might be relatively large: all adult males, a whole country, or all people with type 2 diabetes. Unless the target population is very small, measuring the entire target population or even randomly sampling from it may be impossible.

Instead, a more specific source population (sometimes called a *sampling frame*) should be identified. Ideally, the source population consists of an enumerated list of population members. For example:

- All women with a breast cancer diagnosis in the past 2 years who are indexed in a particular cancer registry
- All members of a professional sports league
- All households within 2 miles of a particular nuclear power plant

In each of these examples, it would be possible for a researcher to acquire or generate a list of all members of the source population. (The list does not have to include the names of the members of the source population. The list might instead include registry identification numbers or street addresses.)

■ 16.3 Sample Populations

Sometimes every person who is listed as a member of the source population will be as
to participate in a study, especially when the source population is small. In this situ
tion, the source population is the same as the sample population. However, a source
population is often much larger than the sample size required for a study. In this situation, only a portion of the source population is selected to serve as a sample population.

A variety of methods can be used to select the sample population. If a list of every
individual in the source population is available, a computer program can be used to
select at random the individuals who will be asked to participate. If the sample will
be drawn from an entire city, then cluster sampling can be used to identify at random
whole city blocks for inclusion in the sample population. Alternatively, the sample
population might consist of all residents in the city living on every tenth street that
runs north to south. Examples of these types of probability-based samples are shown
in FIGURE 16-2.

Sometimes a non-probability-based *convenience population* can be selected based
on the ease of access to those individuals, schools, or communities. Convenience sampling must always be used with caution. Convenient sample populations are often systematically different than the communities they are intended to represent.

No matter which sampling method is used, the goal is to end up with a sample
population that is representative of the source population and, ideally, of the target population too. If random sampling is intended, the researcher needs to avoid the *nonrandom-sampling bias* that could occur if each individual in the source population
does not have an equal chance of being selected for the sample population. If non-
probability sampling (convenience sampling) is used, the researcher must avoid the
ascertainment bias that can occur if the convenience sample is not representative of the
source or target population as a whole. These and many other potential sources of
bias can be eliminated or minimized with careful planning.

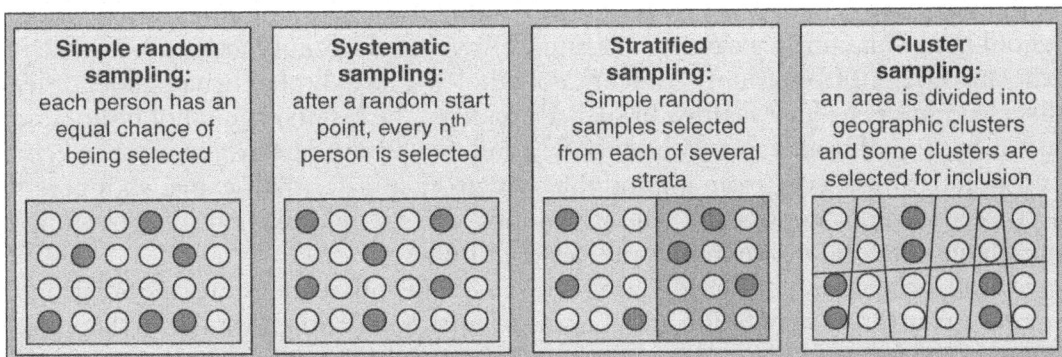

Simple random sampling: each person has an equal chance of being selected	Systematic sampling: after a random start point, every n^{th} person is selected	Stratified sampling: Simple random samples selected from each of several strata	Cluster sampling: an area is divided into geographic clusters and some clusters are selected for inclusion

FIGURE 16-2 Examples of Types of Probability Sampling

◼ 16.4 Study Populations

The individuals identified as the sample population will later be asked to participate in the study. The study population will consist of the members of the sample population who can be located, who consent to participation, and who meet all eligibility criteria. A 100% participation rate is extremely rare. At least some of the individuals in the source population will ignore an invitation to participate. Some who respond to the invitation will choose not to participate. Others will turn out to be ineligible because they do not meet the inclusion criteria. A low response rate may result in *nonresponse bias* if the members of the sample population who agree to be in the study are systematically different from nonparticipants. However, a less than 100% participation rate is usually not a problem as long as the researcher:

- Uses suitable and carefully explained sampling methods.
- Takes appropriate steps to maximize the participation rate.
- Recruits an adequately large sample size. (Chapter 17 explains how to estimate the sample size required.)
- Reports the number of potential participants at each stage.

◼ 16.5 Populations for Cross-Sectional Surveys

In a cross-sectional survey, the source population must be representative of the target population, and the sample population must be representative of the source population. The goal of most cross-sectional surveys is to describe a specific target population accurately. The results of these surveys are often used to make important resource and policy decisions.

Convenience samples rarely result in a study population that is representative of the target population. For example, suppose the goal is to quantify the prevalence of tobacco use in all high school students in a county. Designating only one high school as the source population is not sufficient (FIGURE 16-3). Working intensely with one school might maximize participation rates. However, the school may enroll students who are different from county students as a whole—more rural or urban, more or less diverse, or more or less wealthy. In such a situation, the results would not be an accurate reflection of health across the county. Similarly, recruiting participants for a general population survey from among the spectators at a football game, shoppers in a grocery store, or donors at a volunteer blood drive would likely result in a sample population that did not represent the target population.

Ideally, the researcher needs some way to confirm that the source population is similar to the target population and that the sample population is similar to the source population. For example, the sample population for the survey in Figure 16-3 can be checked to see whether it yields a proportion of students by grade and sex that is sim-

Target population	Source population	Sample population
High school students in North County	All high school students in North County	All students in 20% of homerooms in all high schools in North County

Study approach	Cross-sectional survey
Study question	What proportion of high school students in North County smoke cigarettes?
Study method	Participants will complete their own paper-based questionnaires.
Target population	Students in grades 9–12 in North County
Source population	All students enrolled in any of the 14 high schools in North County
Source population list	A list of the number of students in each homeroom provided by each high school
Sample population	Based on estimated sample size requirements, 20% of homerooms will be randomly selected from the lists provided, and all students in these homerooms will be asked to participate.
Study population	Eligible individuals from the sample population who agree to participate
Confidentiality	No student names will ever be provided to researchers; surveys will be anonymous.

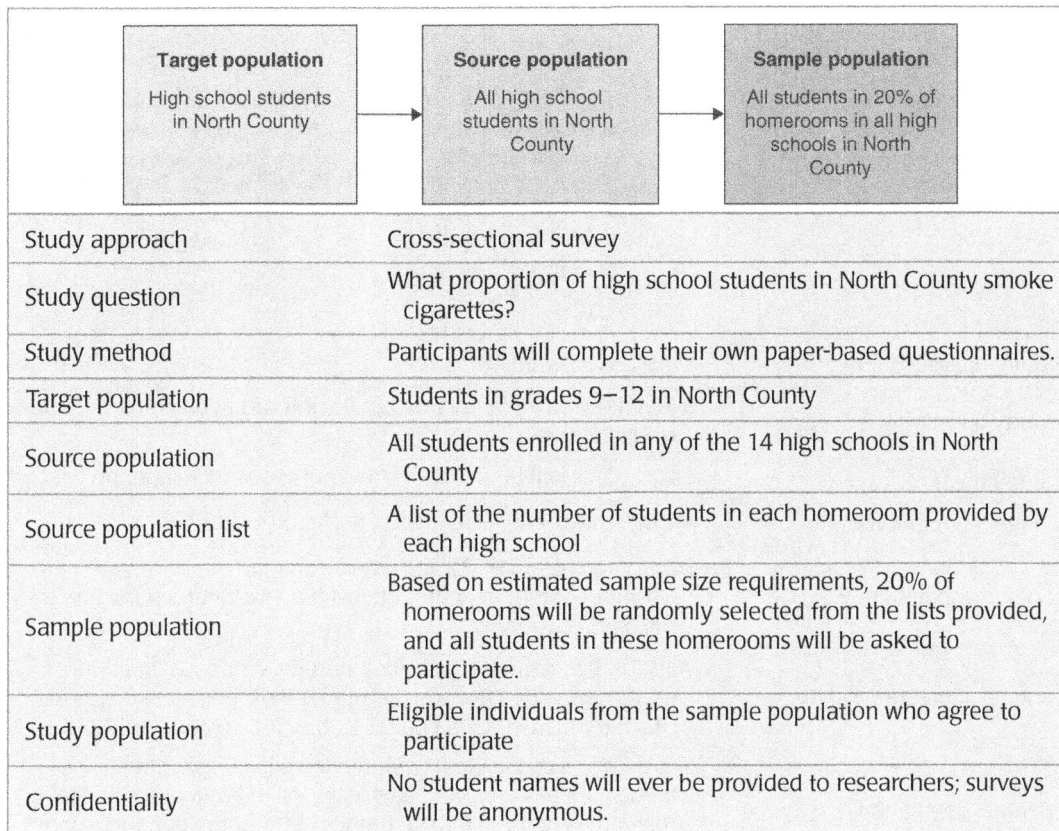

FIGURE 16-3 Population Example for a Cross-Sectional Survey

ilar to the proportions in the source county as a whole. Similarly, the sample population for a survey of the general public should reflect the demographics of the target population in the most recent population census.

16.6 Populations for Case-Control Studies

In identifying possible participants for a case-control study, the first step is to find an appropriate and available source of cases. All cases must have the same disease, disability, or other health-related condition. The study's *case definition* should be very clear about the characteristics, signs, and symptoms that must be present or absent for an individual to be categorized as a case. For example, a researcher may want to select

Target population U.S. women ages 70–79 years	**Source population** All women ages 70–79 years admitted to St. Luke's Hospital System in Center City with an incident hip fracture in the past 12 months and their friends → **Sample population** All women ages 70–79 years admitted to St. Luke's Hospital System in Center City with an incident hip fracture in the past 12 months and three friends per case

Study approach	Case-control study
Study question	What are the risk factors for hip fractures in adult women in the United States?
Study method	Participants will be interviewed in person or by telephone.
Target population	Women ages 70–79 living in the United States
Source population	All women ages 70–79 who were admitted to St. Luke's Hospital System in Center City with an incident hip fracture in the past 12 months
Source population list	A list of the hospital registration numbers for each inpatient female age 70–79 whose computer files indicate a diagnosis of a hip fracture (ICD9 code = 820 or ICD10 code = S72.0)
Sample population	All members of the source population will be asked to participate as cases, and each case will be asked to provide the names of three female friends in the same age range who might be able to serve as controls.
Study population	Eligible individuals from the sample population who agree to participate
Confidentiality	Names, addresses, and phone numbers of potential participants will be provided to the researcher so that potential participants can be contacted. Personally identifying information, such as names, addresses, telephone numbers, and social security numbers, will not be included in the file that contains questionnaire responses.

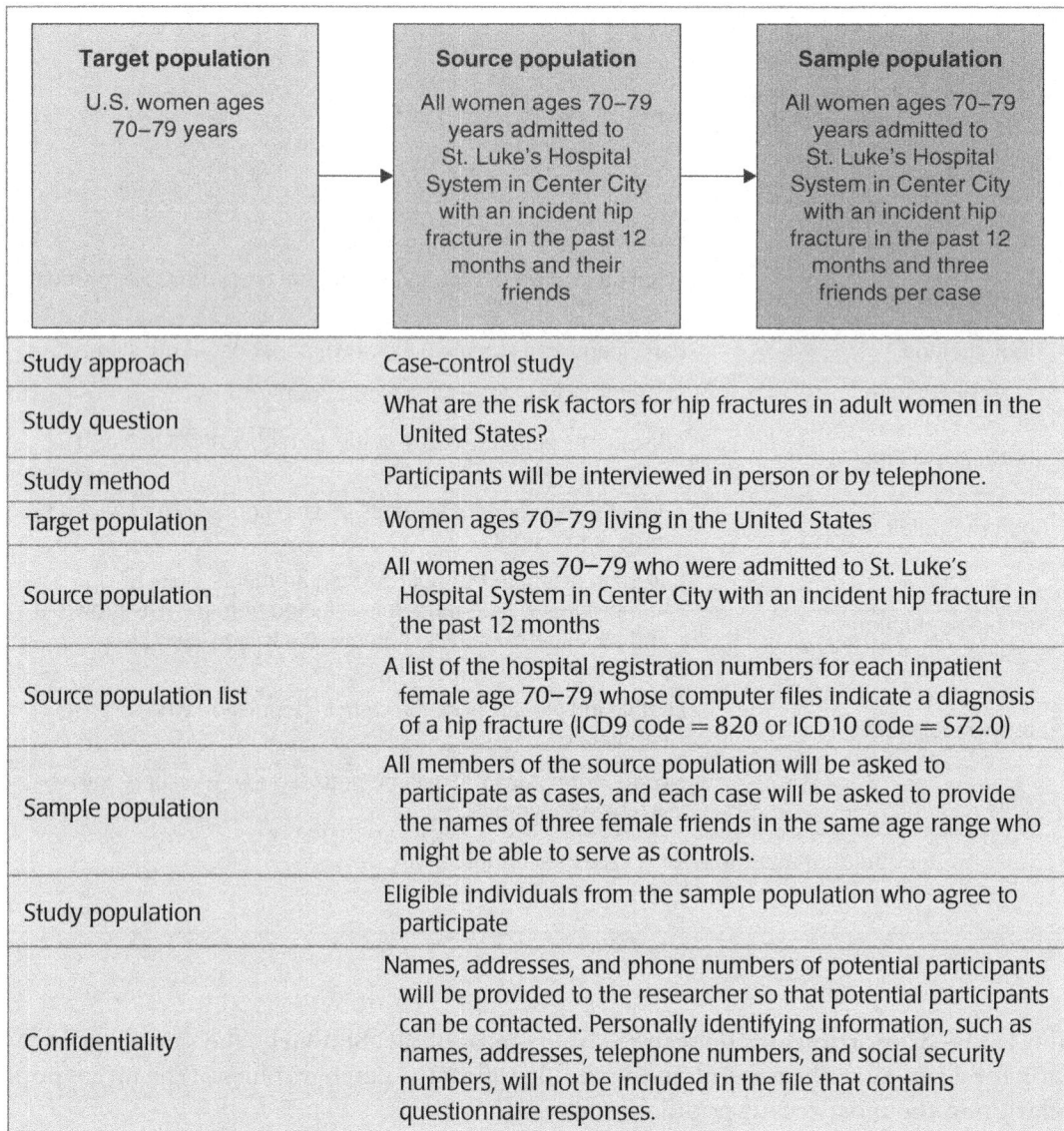

FIGURE 16-4 Population Example for a Case-Control Study

only candidates with advanced disease or, alternatively, may prefer to study only cases with relatively recent onsets of symptoms. The case definition should specify both inclusion and exclusion criteria.

Hospitals, specialty clinics, public health offices, disease support groups, and advocacy organizations may be helpful resources for locating individuals or groups of individuals who are likely to meet the study's case definition. However, care must be taken to ensure that the sample population is not healthier, sicker, or more or less socially connected than the average person who meets the case definition. (Another option may be to use the participants of a large longitudinal cohort study as the source population for both cases and controls. This kind of *nested case-control study* design minimizes recall bias because information about past exposures was collected at the time of the exposure and is not based on participants' memories.)

Once a source of cases is identified, a valid control group must be selected. This is a critical decision. The controls must be similar to the cases in every way except for their disease status. For example, comparing older adult women to teenage boys, comparing people with chronic heart disease to marathon runners, or comparing big-city businessmen to men who are subsistence farmers would not be valid. All cases and all controls must meet the same eligibility criteria except for the ones relating to disease status. (Having both a case definition and a control definition is helpful so that borderline cases are excluded from serving as either cases or controls.) Thus, a study that targets septuagenarian women should require both cases and controls to be women in their 70s (FIGURE 16-4). A study examining chronic disease should choose a control population representative of the general public, not a population that is unusually physically active. And cases and controls for any one study should be drawn from similar geographic and demographic populations.

Controls can be drawn from many different types of source populations. For some hospital-based studies, it may be appropriate to use as controls individuals hospitalized with a condition other than the one being studied. For some population-based studies, random-digit telephone dialing may yield a representative population. Or, because many people will refuse to answer personal questions over the telephone, it may result in a very unrepresentative population. In some situations, friends or family members of the cases may be the best choice because they are likely to have similar backgrounds. When making this important decision, the researcher should consult a reference that specifically addresses the selection of appropriate participants for case-control studies, including the possibilities for matching cases to controls.

■ 16.7 Populations for Cohort Studies

Identifying source and sample populations for a longitudinal cohort study is fairly similar to identifying these populations for a cross-sectional survey (FIGURE 16-5). There are some added concerns about needing to recruit a stable study population in order to retain as many participants as possible for the duration of the study. For cohort studies that seek to compare exposed and unexposed populations, identifying exposed and unexposed participants is similar to the steps for identifying cases and controls for a case-control study.

Target population	**Source population**	**Sample population**
All children with cystic fibrosis (CF) in Canada	All children ages 2–12 years who were patients of the CF clinic of UCH in the past 12 months	All children ages 2–12 years who were patients of the CF clinic of UCH in the past 12 months

Study approach	Cohort study
Study question	What is the incidence rate for lung infections in children with cystic fibrosis?
Study method	Participants' parents will be asked to log all infections throughout the 2-year prospective study period, and these will be checked against the patients' medical records.
Target population	All children with cystic fibrosis in Canada
Source population	All children ages 2–12 years who were patients of the cystic fibrosis clinic of University Children's Hospital (UCH) in the past 12 months
Source population list	A list of all children ages 2–12 who were examined at the UCH cystic fibrosis clinic in the past 12 months
Sample population	The parents of all individuals in the source population will be asked if they will allow their children to participate in the study.
Study population	Eligible individuals from the sample population whose parents agree to let them participate
Confidentiality	All guidelines and regulations for the protection of patient information will be strictly adhered to, and only essential personnel will have access to patient records.

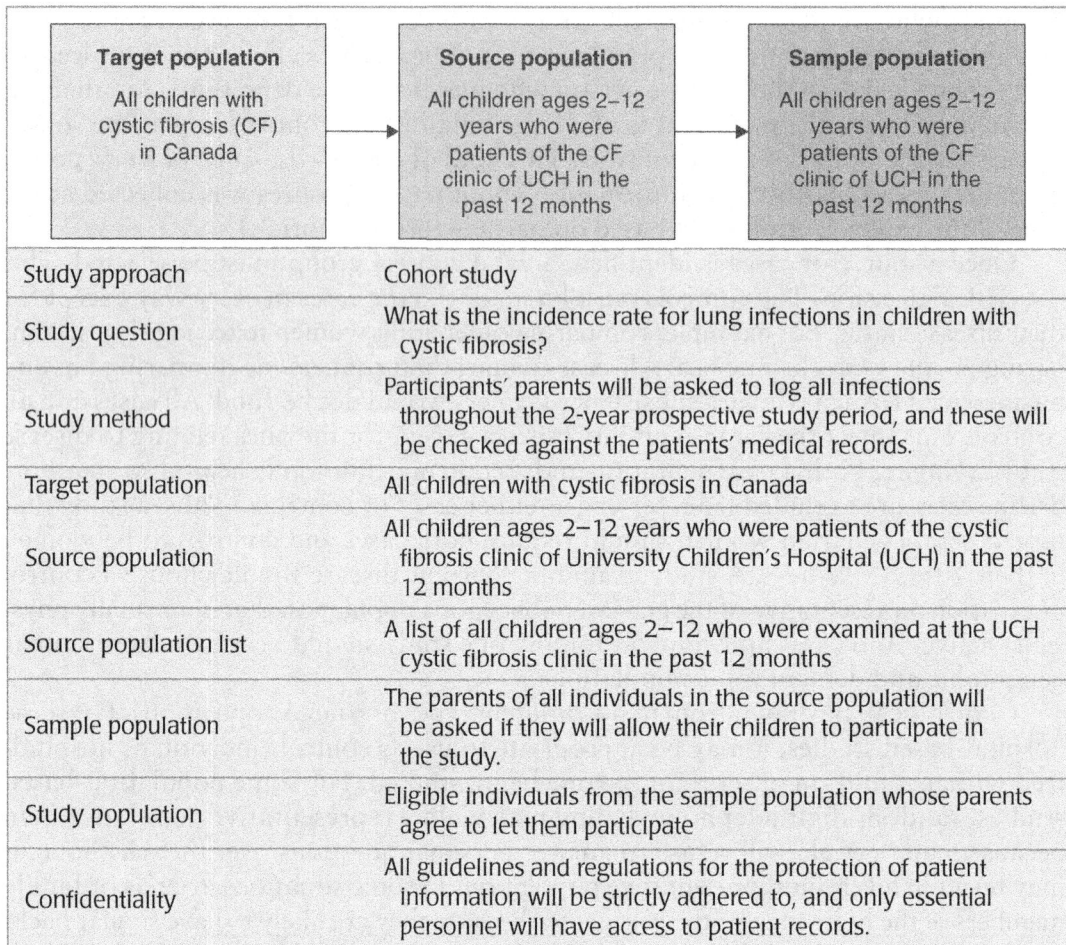

FIGURE 16-5 Population Example for a Cohort Study

◼ 16.8 Populations for Experimental Studies

As is true for cross-sectional surveys, experimental studies require a source population that is reasonably representative of the target population. For example, suppose the goal of an experimental study is to see whether nutritional counseling during the first semester at a residential college prevents weight gain during the first year of college. The researcher has to recruit a reasonable cross-section of the first-year student population (FIGURE 16-6). Some sample selection approaches would likely result in a sample population that was much more concerned about weight than the average first-year

Target population	**Source population**	**Sample population**
First-year students attending primarily residential colleges	All students enrolled in mandatory first-year seminar courses at East State College	A randomly-selected sample of students from the list of enrolled first-year students

Study approach	Experimental study
Study question	Does nutritional counseling during the first semester of college prevent weight gain?
Study method	Half of the participants will be assigned to meet weekly with a nutritionist during their first semester, and half will have no intervention. All participants will complete nutritional assessments during the first and last weeks of the fall and spring semesters of their first year at college.
Target population	First-year students at primarily residential colleges
Source population	All first-year students at East State College
Source population list	A list of all students enrolled in the mandatory first-year seminar class at East State College
Sample population	A randomly selected sample of students from the source population
Study population	Eligible individuals from the sample population who agree to participate
Confidentiality	Nutritional counseling and assessment sessions will be conducted in a private setting, and only essential personnel will have access to participants' records.

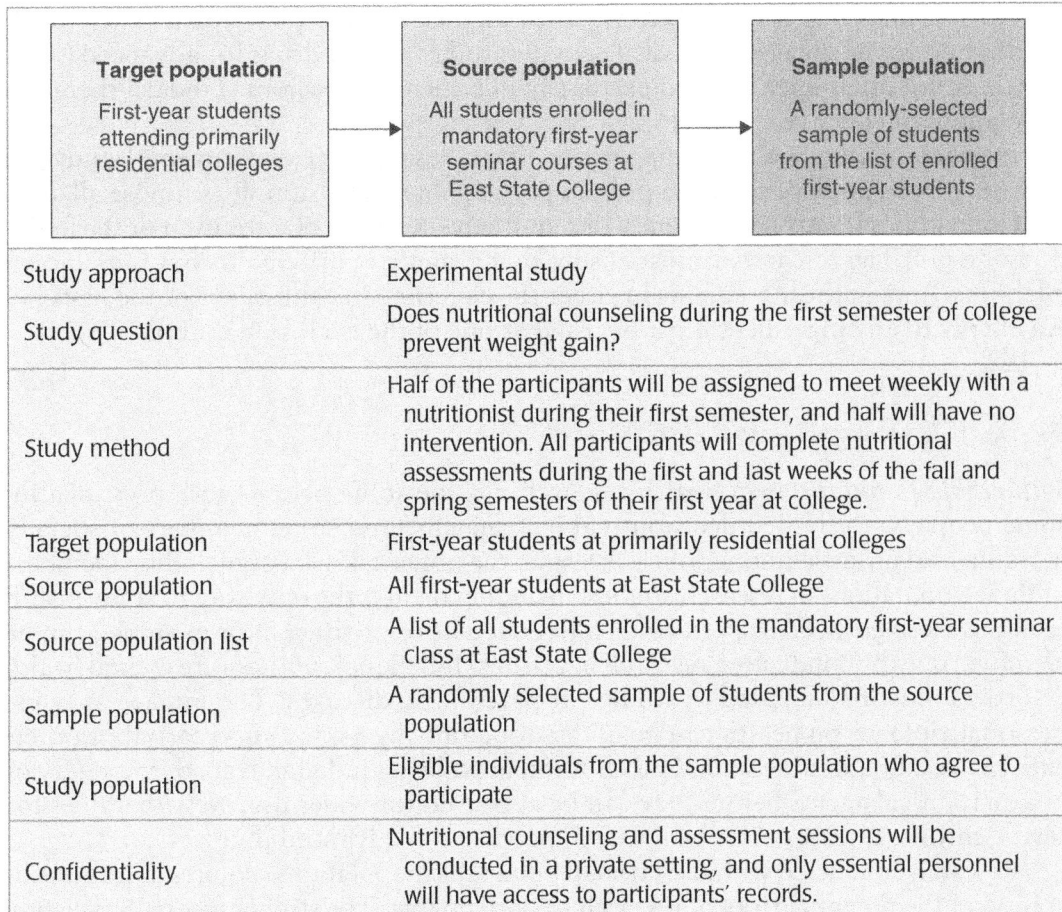

FIGURE 16-6 Population Example for an Experimental Study

student: asking for volunteers, recruiting students enrolled in nutrition classes, or sampling from among student athletes. As a result of any of these methods, both the intervention group, who received nutritional counseling, and the control group, who did not, would be unlikely to gain much weight during the study period. Because there would be no significant difference in weight gain in the intervention and control groups, the intervention would be deemed unsuccessful. Had a more representative study population been recruited, the results might have shown the intervention to be a success.

Some experimental studies require participants to be exposed to potentially risky substances or activities. In such studies, the risk of harm can be reduced by selecting an appropriate source population and defining strict inclusion and exclusion criteria. For example, studies that involve exercise must target potential participants likely to be healthy enough to engage in physical activity. Studies of new drugs for advanced forms of cancer are often open only to extremely ill patients for whom standard therapies have not been effective.

In general, safety is always the top priority in designing an experimental study. All necessary steps must be taken to protect participants. For example, suppose all sampled individuals for an experiment will require the injection of a solution or the ingestion of a pill. The researcher must ensure that potential participants have no known allergies to any of the ingredients in either the experimental substance or the placebo. An allergy to any ingredient must be listed as one of the exclusion criteria.

■ 16.9 Vulnerable Populations

Vulnerable populations in health research include some people with poor health, some people with limited decision-making capacity, and some members of socially marginalized groups, among others. Despite the potential risks of including members of these populations in research studies, including them is the only way to study health issues in these groups. The critical health concerns of prisoners, for example, can be identified only by conducting research in prisons. Individuals with severe mental health disorders must be included in studies of psychiatric diseases. The impact of interpersonal violence on health can be understood only by asking survivors about their experiences. Pregnant women and children must be included in tests of the safety of pharmaceutical agents before they can be approved for wider use. New therapies for severe chronic diseases must be tested in people with advanced illnesses.

Research conducted with members of vulnerable populations requires extra consideration of the potential risks of research to participants. The study must be sufficiently important to justify gathering new data from members of a vulnerable population. The ability of every participant to provide informed consent free from coercion must be assured. (For young children and those with significantly diminished mental capacity, a legally recognized representative must provide consent.) Concerns about the increased risks of adverse effects from study participation must be addressed. For example, people with fragile health may have an elevated risk of injury from physical tests. Those with histories of abuse or mental illness may have a heightened risk of psychological damage from answering questions about sensitive topics. Chapter 21 provides additional information about the requirements of research involving vulnerable populations.

■ 16.10 Community Involvement

Some studies benefit from or require the participation and/or support of whole geographic, cultural, or social communities and their leaders. A cross-sectional survey that will collect information from students may require the permission of school authorities, in addition to the consent of parents and the approval of an ethics committee. A longitudinal study that intends to recruit and follow whole villages will not be a success if formal and informal community leaders and other local representatives are not actively involved in planning, recruitment, and retention. Community-based studies often work best when they use research methods such as those developed for *Community-Based Participatory Research*, or *CBPR*. A clinical study that seeks to enroll participants with an unusual disease may benefit greatly by partnering with an active disease support and advocacy network. These connections should be established early in the research planning process and maintained throughout the data collection period. Also, the results of the study should be shared with partners as soon as they are available.

Primary Studies: Estimating Sample Size

An adequate number of study participants is required to achieve valid and significant results.

■ 17.1 Importance of Sample Size

In a popular children's story, Goldilocks explores the home of three bears. She finds that some of their possessions are too small, some are too big, and some are exactly the right size. Similarly, when determining how many participants are needed for a study to be meaningful, the goal is to recruit just the right number of participants. The right number is based on statistical estimations about how many people are required to answer the study question with a specified level of certainty. If more participants are recruited than are statistically required, resources are wasted, including the time of both the researcher and the participants. If too few participants are recruited, the whole study will be almost worthless because the sample will not have enough statistical power to answer the study question. Few researchers ever have the luxury of worrying about a surplus of participants, but many struggle to recruit a sufficient study population. A shortage can make getting statistically significant results almost impossible.

■ 17.2 Bigger Samples Are Usually Better

There is value in having a large sample size. Large samples from a population are usually better than small ones at yielding a sample mean close to the true population value. For example, suppose that the average (mean) age of 20 people in a total population is 39 years (FIGURE 17-1). If a sample of only 3 people is taken (15% of the total population), there is some possibility that the sample mean will be close to the population mean of 39 years. But there is also a possibility that the sample mean will be distant from the population mean. If a larger sample of 8 people (40% of the total population) is selected from the population, then the sample mean is likely to be fairly close to the population mean.

FIGURE 17-2 shows an alternative display of the sample means that combines the mean age with its 95% confidence interval. A *confidence interval* is a statistical estimate of how close to the population value (in this case, the population mean age) a sample of a particular size is expected to be. When the sample size is small, the sample mean may be quite far from the mean in the total population. This is represented by a wide confidence interval that reaches far from the sample mean. When the sample size is large, the sample mean is expected to be close to the population mean, and the confidence interval will be narrower.

The black dots in the center of each of the five lines in Figure 17-2 represent the five sample means from Figure 17-1. The 95% confidence interval for each sample population is represented by the lines extending from the sample means. The 95% confidence interval is calculated for each sample based on the sample size, the mean

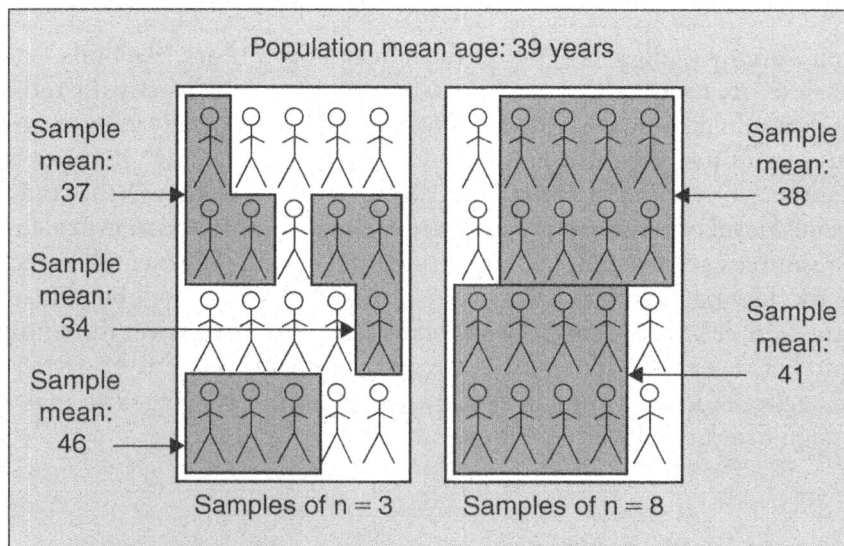

FIGURE 17-1 Sample Size and Means

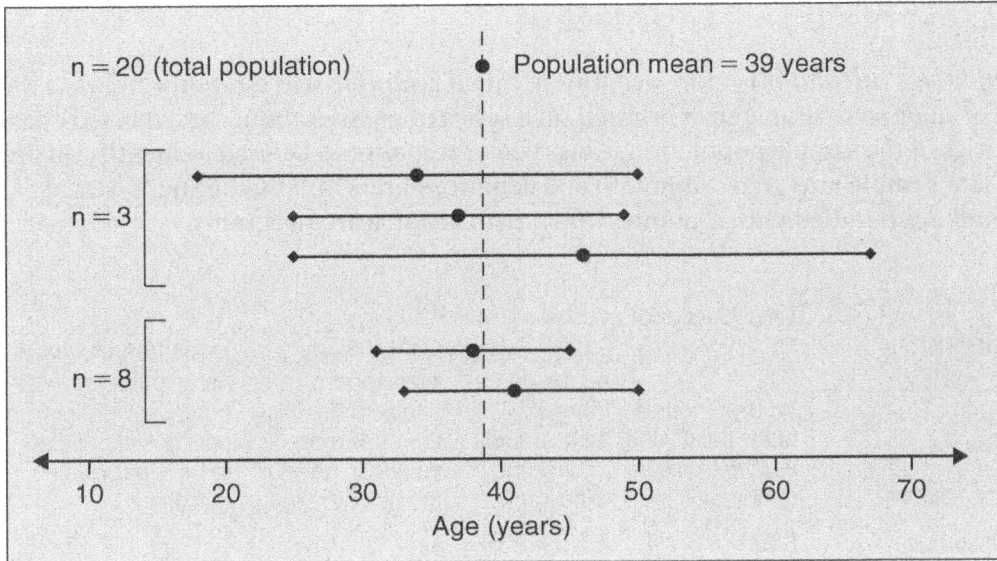

FIGURE 17-2 Larger Samples from a Population Have a Narrower 95% Confidence Interval Than Smaller Samples

age of the sample, and the standard deviation of the sample, which is a measure of how far apart the ages of the individuals in the sample are. For the top line in Figure 17-2, the sample mean is 34 years, and the confidence interval stretches from 18 to 50 years. Based on this sample, a researcher can be 95% confident that the mean in the total population is somewhere between 18 and 50 years. Indeed, the population mean of 39 years is captured in that range. If hundreds of random samples of 3 individuals are drawn from the total population of 20, about 95% of those samples will have a 95% confidence interval that overlaps with the true population mean of 39 years. About 5% of the time, the random sample of 3 individuals will by chance include an unusually young or unusually old set of individuals, and the confidence interval will not overlap with the population mean.

If all 20 people in the total population are included in the analysis, no confidence interval is required; the population mean age will be known exactly. If a sample of 18 of the 20 members of the population is drawn, the sample mean age will be very close to 39 years. The confidence interval will be so narrow that it will hardly extend beyond the dot representing the sample mean. Figure 17-2 shows that larger sample sizes generally result in sample means that are closer to the population mean. Larger sample sizes also have confidence intervals that are narrower than the confidence intervals generated by smaller sample sizes. More generally, larger sample sizes make it more likely that a study will yield statistically significant results.

■ 17.3 Sample Size Estimation

A *sample size calculator* is more accurately called a *sample size estimator* because the range of suggested sample sizes is based on a series of guesses about the expected characteristics of the sample population. This type of tool should be used to identify an appropriate sample size goal. Sample size calculators are available online, often at no cost, and are bundled with a number of statistical software programs.

Characteristic	Cross-Sectional Survey	Case-Control Study	Cohort Study	Experimental Study
Study question	What proportion of the population has the exposure or disease?	Are cases more likely than controls to have the exposure?	Are exposed people more likely than unexposed people to develop the outcome?	Are exposed people more likely than unexposed people to have a favorable outcome?
Population size	5000	—	—	—
Anticipated percentage with exposure or disease	15%	—	—	—
Confidence for anticipated exposure percentage	±3%	—	—	—
Ratio of controls to cases	—	2	—	—
Ratio of unexposed to exposed	—	—	1	1
Anticipated percentage of controls exposed	—	25%	—	—
Anticipated percentage of unexposed with disease or outcome	—	—	10%	70%
OR worth detecting	—	1.5	—	—
RR worth detecting	—	—	1.3	1.25
Confidence level $(1 - \alpha)$	95%	95%	95%	95%
Power $(1 - \beta)$	—	80%	80%	80%
Estimated sample size	**~500**	**~350 cases and 700 controls**	**~1850 exposed and 1850 unexposed**	**~90 exposed and 90 unexposed**

FIGURE 17-3 Examples of Sample Size Calculation

FIGURE 17-3 shows examples of the kinds of inputs that must be provided for various study approaches in order to get a rough estimate of the required number of participants. A best guess must be used for most of these inputs because accurate information will not be available until after the study has been completed. Trying a variety of values for these variables will show that even slight changes in inputs may result in a considerable difference in the sample size estimate. When the level of certainty about inputs is low, erring on the side of a larger sample size is wise.

Also important is that the sample size estimates refer to the study population. Because the participation rate is unlikely to be 100%, the sample population needs to be larger than the number suggested by sample size calculations in order to yield a study population of adequate size.

■ 17.4 Power Estimation

Another way to check for sample size requirements is to work backward from the number of participants likely to be recruited to see whether that sample size provides adequate statistical power for the study design. *Power* is related to the ability of a statistical test to detect significant differences in a population when differences really do exist. For example, suppose that there really is a substantial difference in the mean weight of cases and controls in a case-control study or that an exposure in a cohort study is truly a risk factor for the disease outcome of interest. In such situations, a study needs adequate power to detect those meaningful differences or relationships. When differences between means are close to one another or when relative risks and odds ratios have a point estimate close to 1, sample sizes must be especially large to increase detection power.

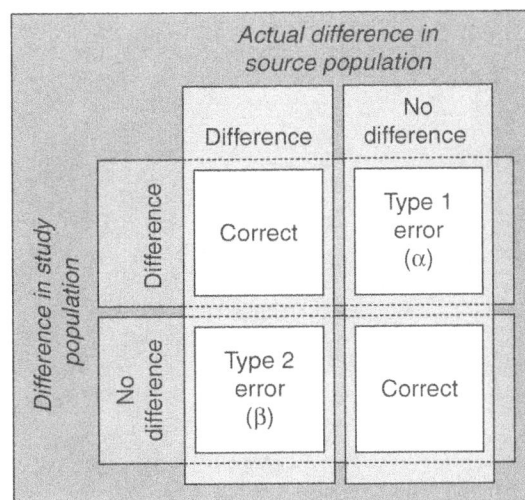

FIGURE 17-4 **Power and Errors**

FIGURE 17-4 illustrates the definition of statistical power. Population-based studies aim to have study populations that reflect their source populations. Sometimes, however, either because of chance or because of a study design flaw (such as too small a sample size), the sample does not capture the true experience of the population. Type 1 errors occur when a study population yields a significant statistical test result when one does not exist in the source population. The probability of a type 1 error is often noted by the Greek letter alpha (α). Most studies aim to have $\alpha = 5\%$, which corresponds to statistical tests using a 95% confidence interval. Type 2 errors occur when a statistical test of data from the study population finds no significant result when one actually exists in the source population. The probability of a type 2 error is often referred to using the Greek letter beta (β). Power is defined as $1 - \beta$. So $\beta = 20\%$ corresponds to power = 80%.

Examples of power estimation for various study approaches are shown in FIGURE 17-5. Like sample size estimates, power estimates require best guesses about the expected findings of the study. The standard expectation is that a study should have a power of 80% or greater. If the power is lower than desired, the easiest way to improve power is usually to increase the sample size.

Characteristic	Cross-Sectional Survey	Case-Control Study	Cohort Study	Experimental Study
Number of exposed	100	—	2500	70
Number of unexposed	250	—	1500	70
Number of cases	—	250	—	—
Number of controls	—	490	—	—
Percentage of exposed with disease or outcome	40%	—	13%	85.7%
Percentage of unexposed with disease or outcome	26%	—	9%	64.3%
Percentage of cases with exposure	—	32%	—	—
Percentage of controls with exposure	—	25.5%	—	—
Confidence level $(1 - \alpha)$	95%	95%	95%	95%
Estimated power $(1 - \beta)$	**~70%**	**~45%**	**~97%**	**~80%**

FIGURE 17-5 Examples of Power Calculation

■ 17.5 Refining the Study Approach

Be prepared to rethink the study approach if the power for the estimated number of participants is not sufficient. For example, if a researcher expects to be able to recruit about 300 participants but the sample size estimates suggest that 870 participants will be required, then the intended study design will not work. In this situation, the study question, study approach, and/or target and source populations must be refined. A new plan must be crafted that is suitable for the sample that the researcher can reasonably expect to recruit.

Primary Studies: Developing a Questionnaire

A questionnaire is a tool for systematically gathering information from study participants. Questionnaires can be designed for self-reporting or as scripts for interviews.

■ 18.1 Questionnaire Design Overview

Questionnaires can be developed for almost any health topic. A good questionnaire is carefully crafted for a specific purpose. Questionnaire design usually works best when it starts with the identification of the general and specific content to be covered by the survey instrument and then progresses to choosing the types of questions and answers for each topic to be assessed. The wording of each question should be checked carefully. The questions within each section and the sections themselves should be in logical order. The formatting of the document should be visually appealing and easy to follow. Prior to its use, the survey instrument has to be pretested and revised as necessary (FIGURE 18-1). This chapter provides details about each step. The researcher should also consult specialty reference manuals for additional information about designing a valid and useful questionnaire for a particular study question.

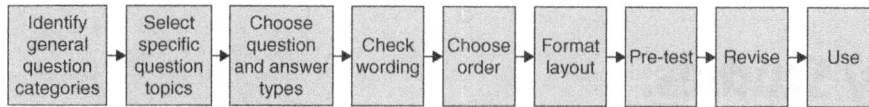

FIGURE 18-1 Questionnaire Design Plan

■ 18.2 Questionnaire Content

The first step in designing a questionnaire is to list the topics that the survey instrument must cover. This list must include the exposure, disease, and population (demographic) areas that are the focus of the study question (FIGURE 18-2). The questionnaire may also include questions about factors that might influence the relationship between exposures and outcomes; these factors are often called *potential confounders*. For example, adults who smoke tobacco products may be more likely than other adults to consume large volumes of alcohol. In a study of the relationship between smoking and liver disease, the use of alcohol could be a potential confounder. Because smokers are more likely than nonsmokers to drink, tobacco users may appear to be at a greater risk of liver disease than nonsmokers, even if the rate of liver disease is the same in smokers who drink as it is in nonsmokers who drink. Asking questions about both tobacco use and alcohol use enables the researcher to statistically adjust for different levels of alcohol use by smokers and nonsmokers and thus to more accurately examine the possible relationship between smoking and liver disease. A thorough search of the literature for studies on similar topics will help in identifying the range of question areas that should be included in the questionnaire.

It is often helpful to start with a list of the main categories of questions to be asked, and then to add detail about the specific topics to be covered. For example, a survey of physical fitness might include sections on demographics, cardiorespiratory fitness, muscle strength, muscle endurance, flexibility, and body composition. (These categories would work equally well for a self-assessment tool and for a laboratory-based assessment tool.) A survey about risk factors for breast cancer might have sections on:

- Sociodemographics (such as age, ethnicity, education level, and income)
- Family health history
- Personal health history (such as previous diagnoses of benign breast diseases and the date of the last screening mammogram)
- Reproductive history (including questions about gravidity, characteristics of menstrual cycles, and use of hormones)
- Lifestyle factors (such as alcohol use, exercise history, and working the night shift)

The questionnaire must include questions confirming that participants meet the eligibility criteria for the study. For example, if only currently registered students are

Demographics	Key exposures	Key diseases/ outcomes	Related exposures and outcomes

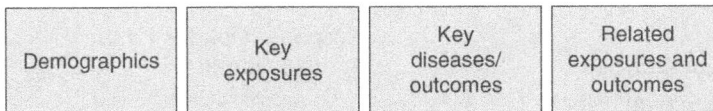

FIGURE 18-2 **Question Areas**

supposed to participate in a university-based cross-sectional survey, one of the first questions should be about enrollment status.

The questionnaire must also be able to accurately place participants into key categories. For example, in case-control studies, researchers need to ask questions that allow them to confirm that all cases meet the case definition. Cohort studies require a series of questions about exposures and about disease status. The answers to these questions must provide evidence that participants did not have the disease outcome of interest at the start of the observation period.

A final consideration is the length of the survey. A survey that is too short will miss potentially crucial information. A survey that is too long may yield a low response rate.

■ 18.3 Types of Questions

After determining the broad categories of questions and the specific topics to be addressed in each section, the next step is to decide which types of questions are appropriate. Each question topic should be assigned a specific type of question, such as a date question or a yes/no question. Examples of these and other question types are shown in FIGURE 18-3. Question types lend themselves to particular types of analysis. It may be helpful to refer to Figure 26-2, which has additional information about variable types.

Close-ended questions, which allow a limited number of possible answers, are usually easier to statistically analyze than *open-ended*, or *free-response*, questions. The main limitation of close-ended questions is that they may force respondents to select answers that do not truly express their status or opinions. Open-ended questions allow participants to explain their selections and qualify their responses, to give multiple answers, and to provide responses not anticipated by the researchers. However, open-ended questions take longer to ask and answer, and they may result in irrelevant answers. Recoding free-response answers into objective and meaningful categories for statistical analysis is often time-consuming and difficult. Open-ended questions are often most useful when they are used to get initial impressions or to clarify responses to close-ended questions.

Close-ended questions come in a variety of formats, including date and time variables (which can be used to calculate the length of time between events), numeric variables, and categorical variables.

Type	Sample Question	Response Options for the Sample Question
Date	What is your birth date?	_ _ - _ _ - _ _ _ _ m m - d d - y y y y
Numeric	What is your height without shoes (rounded to the nearest half inch)?	_ _ . _ inches
Yes/no	During your lifetime, have you smoked more than 100 cigarettes?	☐ Yes ☐ No
Categorical/ multiple-choice: nominal (no rank)	What is your sex?	☐ Female ☐ Male
	What is your favorite type of film?	☐ Action/drama ☐ Comedy/musical ☐ Documentary ☐ Other: _____
Categorical/ multiple-choice: ordinal (ranked)	What is the highest level of education you have completed?	☐ Less than high school ☐ High school ☐ Some college but no degree ☐ College degree or more advanced
	How much do you agree with this statement: "No matter how much I exercise, I will not be able to lose weight."	☐ Strongly disagree ☐ Disagree ☐ Neutral ☐ Agree ☐ Strongly agree
	On a scale of 1 to 5, with 1 meaning poor and 5 meaning excellent, how would you rate your hearing (without the use of a hearing aid)?	Poor——————Excellent ☐ 1 ☐ 2 ☐ 3 ☐ 4 ☐ 5
Paired-comparisons	Do you prefer to drink coffee or tea?	☐ I prefer coffee ☐ I prefer tea ☐ I like coffee and tea equally ☐ I do not drink coffee or tea
Rank-ordering	List the following four political issues in order from most important to you (1) to least important to you (4): crime/safety, environment/energy, foreign policy/defense, taxes/revenue	Number from 1 (most important) to 4 (least important): ___ Crime/safety ___ Environment/energy ___ Foreign policy/defense ___ Taxes/revenue
Open-ended/ free-response	What is your biggest personal health concern at present?	_____ _____

FIGURE 18-3 Examples of Types of Questions

Categorical variables can have as few as two options (called *dichotomous variables*), like yes/no or male/female, or they can have dozens of possible answers. Categorical variables can also be ranked (*ordinal*) or unordered (*nominal*). Ordinal responses have an inherent order, and nominal responses do not have any built-in order. For example, a question about educational level is ordinal because some levels of education involve more years of school than other levels do. A question about occupational category is nominal because there is no obvious way to rank occupations as diverse as plumbing, farming, teaching, nursing, sales, and law.

Less used question types include paired-comparisons and rank-ordering questions.

■ 18.4 Anonymity

Many questions can be asked in more than one valid way. The researcher must decide which question type is most appropriate and will best protect participants' anonymity. For example, participants' ages can be ascertained in a number of ways. One is by asking for the date of birth and calculating the number of years between the birthdate and the interview or survey date. However, asking for such specific personal information may raise concerns about anonymity because birth dates could be personal identifiers in a small population. Additionally, the fear of providing identifying information may mean that many participants will skip the question entirely. Some may even drop out of the study rather than provide a birthdate. To protect participants and reduce fears about privacy, the researcher could ask for each participant's current age in years rather than for a date of birth. Even then, age in years could reveal the identity of some individuals in the study population. In surveys of college students, for instance, most participants will fall into a fairly narrow age range; much younger or older students will stand out. In such cases, it might be best simply to ask participants to indicate which age range they belong to (such as ≤20, 21–29, or ≥30).

Similar decisions must be made about each component of the questionnaire that could link participants to their answers. If a name, an address, a birthdate, or other information could link a participant to the study, then there must be a solid plan in place for protecting the privacy of participants and the confidentiality of the information they share (see Chapter 21).

■ 18.5 Types of Responses

Once the types of questions have been selected, a decision must be made about the kinds of responses that are appropriate for the question.

- For numeric responses, the question should state exactly how specific the answers should be. Should height be reported to the nearest inch, to the nearest half inch, to the nearest quarter inch, or to the nearest centimeter?

- For categorical questions, the response categories should be listed. Sometimes an "other" category should be included so that respondents can fill in their own answers if none of the listed responses is applicable. Consider all possible responses for each question, and include as many as needed.
- For ranked questions, decisions must be made about how many entries to include on the scale and whether there will be a neutral option. Most scales with a neutral option list 5 to 7 categories; most scales without a neutral option list 4 or 6 categories. Sample response scales are shown in FIGURE 18-4.

For self-report surveys, a decision must also be made about whether to add a category for "not applicable" or "do not know." For questionnaires to be used as scripts, a "refused to answer" category is needed. Other examples of these types of alternate responses are "no opinion," "not sure," "hard to say," "no answer," "I prefer not to answer," "I do not understand," and "I forget."

Some variables require a definitive answer, so the option for skipping a response might be removed. For example, for many surveys, knowing whether the participant is female or male is important. Most people can answer that question very easily, so an "I do not know" response is not required. However, for a question like "When was the last time you had your blood sugar levels tested?" it may be important to know whether a person is uncertain about the answer. That uncertainty is a valid and interesting response. Neglecting to list "I do not know" as a possible response would force many people to choose an answer they were not sure about. This may hide important information. It may also lead to systematic inaccuracies in the data. For example, information bias may occur if participants who do not know the answer to a question systematically default to providing the answer they assume the researcher wants to hear.

Strongly disagree	Disagree	Neutral	Agree	Strongly agree
Dissatisfied	Somewhat dissatisfied	Neutral	Somewhat satisfied	Satisfied
Very negative	Somewhat negative	Neither negative nor positive	Somewhat positive	Very positive
Poor	Fair	Good	Very good	Excellent
None	Few	Some	Many	Very many
Not at all important	Not too important	Somewhat important	Very important	Extremely important

FIGURE 18-4 **Examples of Responses for Ranked Questions**

■ 18.6 Wording of Questions

After drafting the questionnaire, check each question for clarity.

- Does each question ask what it is intended to ask?
- Is the language of each question clear and neutral?
- Will members of the study population understand the language?
- Is the question sensitive to potential cultural issues related to language?

Also check to be sure that the responses are carefully worded.

- Is the choice of response clear?
- For scaled questions, is the rank order clear? (For example, is it clear that 1 is "strongly disagree" and 5 is "strongly agree"? Or, alternatively, that 1 is "excellent" and 7 is "poor"?)
- For questions with unranked categories, is the order of possible responses alphabetical or otherwise neutral?

FIGURE 18-5 lists examples of potential problems with questions, including problems related to language, content, and responses.

Problem	Example	Problem with the Example
Big words/jargon	Have you ever had a myocardial infarction?	Participants may not know that a "myocardial infarction" is a fancy name for a heart attack.
Undefined abbreviations	Have you ever been told that you have BPH?	Participants may not know that BPH is short for benign prostatic hypertrophy or that BPH means an enlarged prostate.
Ambiguous meanings	What kind of house do you live in?	Without seeing a list of appropriate responses, it is not clear if the answer should be "an apartment," "a rental," "a split-level duplex," or "a single-family home."
Vagueness	Do you exercise regularly?	"Regularly" is not clear. A person who exercises most days of each week might assume that "regularly" means daily and say "no." Another person who exercises once a month may consider that regular. It would be better to ask "In a typical week, how many days do you exercise for at least 30 minutes?"

FIGURE 18-5 Problems to Avoid

Problem	Example	Problem with the Example
Double negatives	I did not find this visit with my doctor to be unpleasant. ☐ Disagree ☐ Neutral ☐ Agree	The wording of this question makes it hard to figure out whether a person who was satisfied with a visit should agree or disagree.
Faulty assumptions	Do your gums bleed during regular dental cleanings? ☐ Yes ☐ No	The question assumes that everyone has routine dental cleanings. If "I do not visit the dentist" is not an answer option, a person who does not have dental cleanings is forced to answer no.
Two-in-one	Do you exercise at least 3 times a week and eat a healthy diet? ☐ Yes ☐ No	Combines two separate questions: one for exercise and one for diet.
Impossible to recall accurately	How many servings of carrots did you eat most weeks when you were a child?	Adults will not be able to remember this level of detail about their childhood diets.
Too much detail	List any prescription medications you have taken for 1 month or longer in the past 10 years.	Unless the respondent has had very few prescriptions, answering this question is impossible without looking up medical records.
Sensitive questions	Have you ever hit, scratched, bruised, or otherwise physically injured an intimate partner?	This question is unlikely to be answered truthfully if the response should be yes, and it may raise concerns about confidentiality and potential legal requirements for reporting abuse.
Hypothetical questions	Have you ever thought that you would like to lose 10 or more pounds?	Anyone could have felt this at some point in time, but the question does not clarify whether this is a long-term longing or a thought that crossed the respondent's mind for the first time upon reading the question.
Leading questions	What is your impression of the quality of work done by the dedicated public servants who work at the county health department?	This question clearly intends to lead respondents toward a positive answer (and may unintentionally have the opposite effect).

FIGURE 18-5 (continued)

Problem	Example	Problem with the Example
Leading answers	What is your impression about the quality of services provided by Center City Hospital? ☐ Fair ☐ Good ☐ Great ☐ Excellent	This question's response options clearly are intended to lead to a positive response; there is no "poor" option.
Answers with a poor scale	How many hours a week do you watch television? ☐ 0 ☐ 1–3 ☐ 4–7 ☐ 8 or more	Even though most people watch more than 1 hour of television daily, which would put them in the "8 or more" response category, they may not want to choose an "extreme" answer. Their inaccurate responses will lead to a false report. Alternatively, these response options may cause respondents to misread the question as how many hours a *day* they watch television.
Lack of specificity	What is your income?	It is not clear if income refers to earnings per hour, week, month, or year, or whether it refers to pre- or post-tax income.
Missing answer options	What color are your eyes? ☐ Brown ☐ Blue	Many possible eye colors are missing.
Overlapping answer options	In a typical week, how many days do you eat fish? ☐ 0 ☐ 1–3 ☐ 3–5 ☐ 5–7	Participants who eat fish 3 days a week or 5 days a week will not know which response to select.

FIGURE 18-5 (continued)

■ 18.7 Order of Questions

Many questionnaires start with easy or at least general questions before moving to more difficult or sensitive questions. The questions should be in an order that flows naturally from one topic to another, and similar questions should be grouped. Sometimes similar questions with similar response types can be best asked consecutively. Other times, it is better to mix up such questions to prevent *habituation*. This occurs when respondents have given the same answer to so many questions in a row ("agree . . . agree . . . agree . . .") that they continue to reply with the same response because it has become routine. Think carefully about how previous questions could taint the answers to later ones. For example, once a participant has considered a variety of options, he or she can no longer provide an unbiased first impression. Thus, the researcher may want to order questions about impressions this way:

- First, an open-ended question to garner a first impression from participants: "What do you do most often when _____?"
- Second, a series of yes/no questions to clarify beliefs and practices: "Do you ever _____?"
- Last, a concluding, open-ended question to allow participants to express final impressions: "Now that you have considered the possibilities, what would you say you do most often when _____?"

■ 18.8 Layout and Formatting

The next step in questionnaire design is formatting the document so that it is organized, easy to read, and easy to record answers on. Use a readable and large font. The answer sheet should clearly indicate where and how responses should be marked. *White space* (blank areas) on the page is helpful. It clearly separates sections and makes the page visually appealing. If necessary, very clear instructions for *skips* should direct interviewers or respondents to jump over sets of nonapplicable questions.

The layout of the survey instrument will vary depending on the mechanism of data collection used. A written survey (FIGURE 18-6) that respondents complete on their own on paper may require a cover letter and instructions about how to indicate answers, such as:

Basic Information			
1. What is today's date?	__ __ - __ __ - __ __ __ __ m m d d y y y y		
2. What is your date of birth?	__ __ - __ __ - __ __ __ __ m m d d y y y y		
3. What is your sex?	☐ Female	☐ Male	
Health History (*Check one answer box for each question.*)			
4. Have you ever been diagnosed with breast cancer?	☐ Yes	☐ No	→ *If No, then skip to question 7.*
5. Have you had a mastectomy (either partial or complete)?	☐ Yes	☐ No	

FIGURE 18-6 **Example of a Self-Reported Questionnaire**

Fill in today's date.	__ __ - __ __ - __ __ __ __ mm dd y y y y	
Read: *Thank you for agreeing to participate in this health study. I'm going to start by asking you some basic questions.*		
1. What is your date of birth?	__ __ - __ __ - __ __ __ __ mm dd y y y y	☐ Refused to answer
2. What is your sex: female or male?	☐ Female ☐ Male	
Read: *Now I'm going to ask you a few questions about your medical history.*		
3. Have you ever been diagnosed with breast cancer?	☐ Yes ☐ No	→ *If **No**, then skip to question 6.*
4. Have you had a mastectomy (either partial or complete)?	☐ Yes ☐ No	☐ Refused to answer

FIGURE 18-7 Example of a Telephone Interview Script (for the same questions as in Figure 18-6)

- "Select the one answer that best describes you."
- "Fill in the oval in front of your answer completely using blue or black ink."
- "Circle all options that apply to you."
- "Write your answer in block capital letters, as shown in the example below."

An Internet-based survey has the benefit of allowing the researcher to build skips into the program so that irrelevant questions do not even appear on the screen. Computer-based surveys can also force a person to give an answer to one or more questions before the next set of questions is revealed. However, a problem can result from making some fields required. Required fields force a person who does not want to provide an answer to quit the survey at that question.

In an oral survey (FIGURE 18-7), the interviewer will read the questions to the respondent and note the answers given. In addition to the questions, it will require a script that has an opening statement, transitions between sections of the survey, and closing sentences. The questionnaire must clearly indicate the sections to be read aloud, the spaces for recording responses, and other instructions.

After formatting, the document should be carefully checked for grammatical errors, misspellings, missing questions, gaps in logic, unclear instructions, formatting errors, and other organizational issues. If the questionnaire appears to be too long, it may be helpful to cut some questions.

■ 18.9 Validation

A valid questionnaire (or other assessment tool) measures what it was intended to measure in the population being assessed. One way to seek validity is to include survey questions or modules that are identical to the ones used in previous research projects. However, access to survey questions is often not possible in the health sciences. Copies of questionnaires are almost never included in published papers and are only rarely posted on researchers' websites. As a result, new research projects usually require the development and testing of a completely new survey instrument. Pilot testing of the new questionnaire is essential for the development of a valid and useful tool.

■ 18.10 Commercial Research Tools

Several widely used and validated tests are available to researchers, such as:

- For psychological status: the Beck Depression Inventory and the General Health Questionnaire (GHQ)
- For cognition: the Mini-Mental State Examination (MMSE)
- For health-related quality of life: the SF-36 and SF-12

The Buros Institute's *Mental Measurements Yearbook* provides reviews of thousands of available tools used in psychological and educational assessment. Some of these tools are free of charge, but most are commercial products that require payment for use. For some instruments provided at no charge, researchers have to pay to have the results scored and validated against previous users of the survey instrument.

■ 18.11 Translation

Translation of the survey instrument into one or more additional languages may be necessary if the sample population contains speakers of more than one language. (Translation may also be required when an ethics review committee may require materials to be presented in the committee's preferred language as well as in the language of the sample population.) Check to be sure that the translated version expresses the same meaning as the original survey. Accuracy may require the rephrasing of whole sentences, not just direct word-for-word translations.

One way to ensure that the correct meaning is being conveyed is to use *back translation*, or *double translation*. One person translates the questionnaire from the original language to a new language; a second person then translates the survey instrument in the new language back into the original language. A comparison of the original version of the survey with the back-translated version will reveal where the second-language translation does not match the intended meaning of the original version. A second approach is to have two translators independently translate the survey instrument from the original to the new language. Then the two translations are compared to see which words and phrases best convey the precise meaning and complexity of the original questionnaire.

■ 18.12 Pilot Testing

A *pilot test*, or *pretest*, of the questionnaire is helpful for checking, among other issues:

- The wording and clarity of the questions.
- The order of the questions.
- The ability and willingness of participants to answer the questions.
- The responses given, and whether the responses match the intended types of responses.
- The amount of time it takes to complete the survey.

The researcher should ask several volunteers to help with the pilot test. They should be from the target population, meet the eligibility criteria for the study (in terms of age, disease status, or other key factors), but not be in the sample population. They should be asked to complete the preliminary survey and then provide feedback about content, clarity, layout, timing, and other factors. They can provide feedback individually or in a focus group.

The survey instrument should be revised based on these observations. Several rounds of pilot testing may be required to develop a sound survey instrument.

Primary Studies: Surveys and Interviews

Most primary studies collect data from individual participants using an interview method or a self-administered questionnaire. Self-reported surveys are usually the least costly and least time-consuming way to gather information. However, interviews may allow for more detailed information to be gathered and can be accompanied by laboratory and other tests.

■ 19.1 Interviews Versus Self-Administered Surveys

The first decision to make about data collection is whether to have a member of the research team interview participants or to have participants record their own answers (FIGURE 19-1). *Interviews* may be conducted in person or via the telephone. The primary advantage of an interview is that trained interviewers record the responses, and they can ensure the accuracy and completeness of each questionnaire. *Self-administered surveys* can be completed at a specific research site, such as a workplace or school or hospital, or they can be delivered by mail or the Internet. The key benefits of self-administered questionnaires are that data collection from a large number of participants is cost effective and they may be the best way to get honest answers to sensitive questions.

The most important considerations when deciding which approach to use are the goals of the study and the expectations of the sample population members. Secondary considerations are cost, time, and potential barriers to participation. For example, in terms of cost:

- For interviews, the highest cost is usually personnel.
- For mail surveys, the highest costs are typically photocopying, postage, and data entry.

Interview		Self-administered survey		
A member of the research team asks questions of participants and records their responses		Participants are provided with a set of questions and record their own answers		
In-person (face-to-face) interview	Telephone interview	Completion in presence of researchers	Mail (postal) survey	E-mail/ internet-based survey

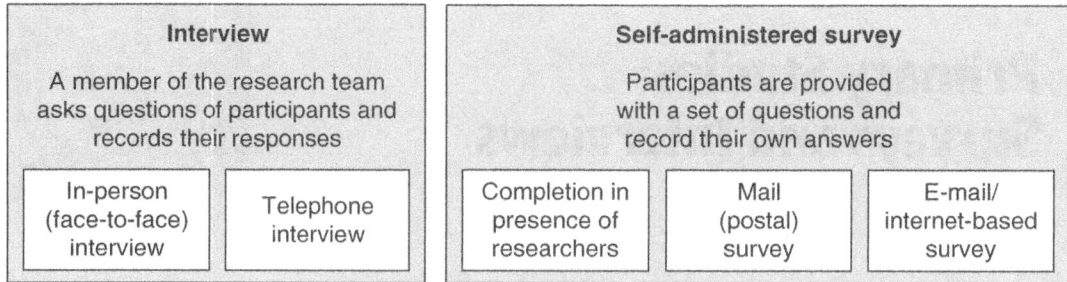

FIGURE 19-1 Examples of Methods for Collecting Data

- For Internet-based surveys, the costs may be relatively low if a free or low-cost survey-hosting Web site is used.

In estimating the cost per participant, consider the likely participation rate. Mailing out 10 surveys may be necessary to receive one completed questionnaire, and the budget and sample size estimates should reflect this expectation.

Time is another consideration. Asking participants to complete their self-administered questionnaires at the same place and time can generate a lot of data quickly. One-on-one interviews may take a considerable amount of time per participant, but all interviews may be able to be scheduled within a relatively short period of time. Mail surveys may trickle in over an extended period of time and make it challenging for a researcher to know when to stop waiting for additional responses to arrive.

The barriers to participation also vary according to the data collection method. Transportation to the interview site may be difficult for some interviewees. Discomfort with the telephone or computer may be a challenge for others.

■ 19.2 Recruiting Methods

Once a data collection method has been selected, the next step is to decide on an effective method for recruiting members of the sample population to be participants in the study. The goal of recruiting is twofold: (1) to recruit as many members of the sample population as possible and (2) to yield a study population that is reasonably representative of the sample population. With regard to the second goal, the researcher should try to find a way to compare the characteristics of participants to those of the source population. For example, the age distribution of the source population can be compared to that of the study population. A statistical test can be used to determine whether the study population skewed old or young or was spot on.

The best method for initiating contact with potential participants is often related to the intended data collection method (FIGURE 19-2).

- If the plan is to interview people in person, the best recruiting method may be to visit potential recruits at work, at school, at home, at a public venue, or at another appropriate location. Alternatively, interviews could be set up by calling sampled individuals or sending a letter or e-mail. (Of course, these methods of contact require the individual's contact information to be known. This would be the case if recruiting patients of a particular clinic or members of a particular organization.)
- If the plan is to interview by telephone, it may be possible to recruit some participants with cold calls. However, the participation rate will likely be higher if a letter of invitation is sent first. (Sending a letter will also allow for the acquisition of signed informed consent forms prior to the interview, if they are required.)

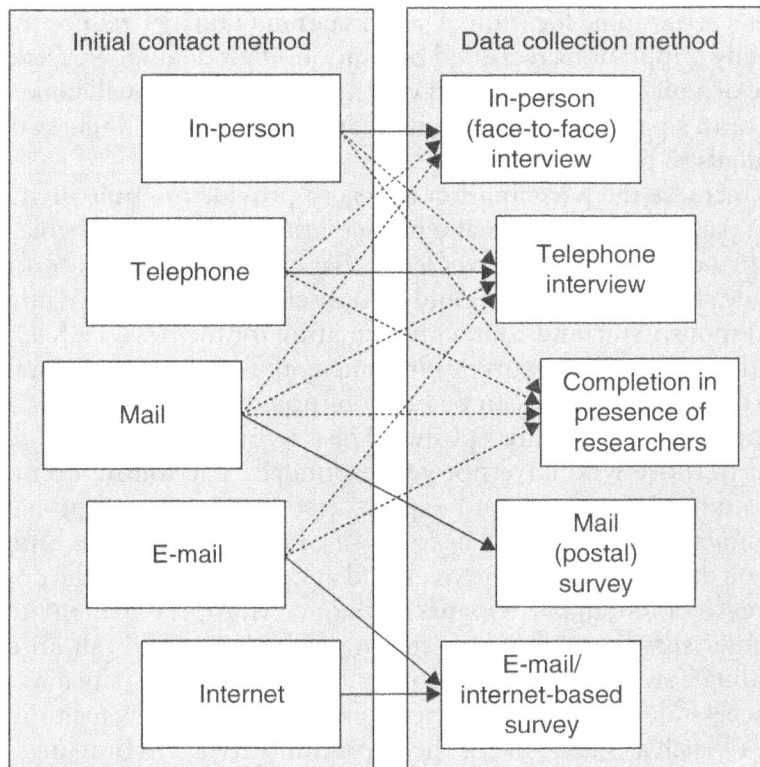

FIGURE 19-2 Examples of Methods for Contacting Members of the Sample Population

- If the plan is to collect data via the Internet, then contacting potential participants via e-mail or a website may be the most effective method.

Participation rates will likely be higher if recruits understand the importance and value of the research project. For example, suppose that the plan is to interview members of a particular organization by phone. The response rate is likely to be highest if interviewers start each phone conversation with potential participants by explaining why the participants are being contacted, how their contact information was acquired, and how completing an interview will assist the organization. The participation rate may be quite high even for unscheduled telephone calls because the importance and relevance of the study is addressed at the start of the call. Support for the study may be even higher still if the study plans are shared ahead of time in an organizational newsletter or via an e-mail to all members.

In contrast, only a few out of every hundred calls made by a *random-digit dialing*—calls to a computer-generated list of unscreened telephone numbers—may yield one person willing to complete a survey. Even then, many willing participants may turn out to be ineligible for the study. Additionally, a growing problem with using random-digit dialing is that mobile phone numbers are often unlisted and are not necessarily indicative of the user's geographic location. These issues may further reduce the representativeness of study populations recruited by random-digit dialing. Nevertheless, using the first minute of a phone call to explain why a particular study will make a difference in the world or to a particular community may increase the willingness of randomly dialed individuals to participate.

Another way to increase the participation rate is to provide multiple invitations and opportunities to participate and to make participation as easy as possible. Mail survey packets should include a concise cover letter that explains the purpose and importance of the survey. The cover letter should also disclose any necessary information such as financial sponsorship and contact information for the research team. The mailed packet should also include the survey instrument and a preaddressed stamped envelope so that the completed survey can be easily returned to the researcher. A few weeks after the initial mailing, a reminder postcard or a second copy of the questionnaire should be sent to those who have not yet responded. The follow-up mailing should reaffirm the study's importance and express gratitude to those who have already returned a completed survey as well as to those who intend to do so. Similarly, multiple phone calls on different days of the week and at different times of the day may have to be made to reach potential participants by phone. Multiple e-mail invitations to complete a computer survey may be required to get recruits to fill out an online questionnaire. Including a step-by-step guide for using the survey Web site may make participation more accessible to those who are uncomfortable with new technologies.

Finally, incentives—such as small gifts or the opportunity to be in a drawing to win an award—may be an effective means of encouraging participation among those invited to be in the study.

■ 19.3 Data Recording Methods

A decision must also be made about how responses will be recorded and when they will be entered into a computer database. There are two basic options (FIGURE 19-3). One is to record the responses on paper and to enter them into a computer database later. The other is to have interviewers or participants enter responses directly into a database.

Paper questionnaires have several benefits. In some environments, they are required for the collection of data from a large number of participants at one time. An example is when all students attending a school need to complete a questionnaire during the same 20-minute period. Paper instruments allow for the easy collection of signatures on informed consent statements, and some researchers value having paper records as a backup. But paper-based surveys have a serious disadvantage: unless somewhat expensive optical scan forms are used, all responses have to be manually entered into a computer at a later time. Data entry is often a very time-consuming process.

The major advantage of computer-assisted surveys is that they eliminate the need for later data entry. They may also simplify the questionnaire by automatically removing any questions not relevant to a particular study participant. For example, they may skip questions specific to females for participants who identify themselves as being male. The main limitation of computer-assisted surveys is that some populations are uncomfortable with computer technology. The members of these population groups will therefore systematically choose not to participate in an Internet-based survey. Discomfort with technology may take other forms. Some interviewees will be distracted by an interviewer who is entering responses into a computer as they give their responses. These individuals might not be similarly bothered by an interviewer with

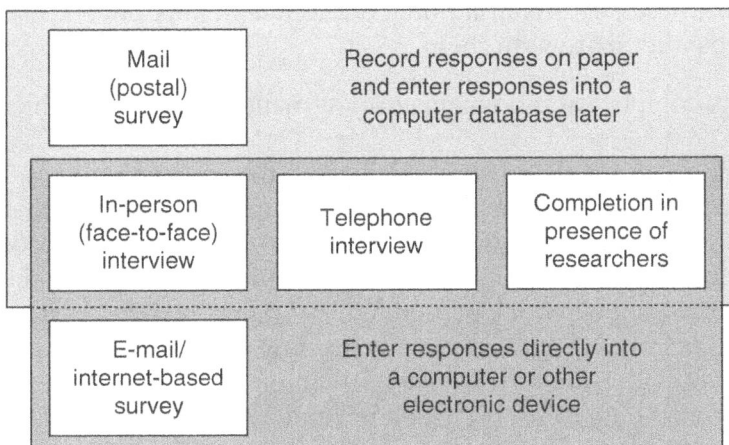

FIGURE 19-3 Methods for Collecting and Recording Survey Data

a clipboard. Additionally, for some studies having a limited number of computer terminals or portable electronic devices so severely limits the number of participants who can complete a survey at any one time that computer use becomes a barrier to project completion.

■ 19.4 Training Interviewers

The interview process should be the same for all participants in a study, whether they are being interviewed in-person or by telephone interview. Uniformity is easiest to accomplish when all interviewers are provided with the tools they need to follow a standardized set of procedures. All interviewers should undergo role-specific training and have an opportunity to practice their interview skills. Each interviewer should be given a comprehensive interviewer handbook that provides information about the purpose of the study, details about interview logistics, an annotated script for the interview, and annotated copies of all study forms. The training and handbook should:

- Explain the interview process step-by-step.
- Specify exactly how to ask questions and record responses.
- Identify any prompts or follow-up questions that the interviewer needs to use.
- Provide preset checklists for managing problems during an interview.

All of this information should be contained in the study protocol.

Interviewers usually feel more prepared for their role after attending one or more training sessions. Facilitators often begin training sessions by:

- Explaining the purpose of the research project.
- Emphasizing the importance of strictly following the procedures spelled out in the interviewer handbook.
- Making clear the absolute necessity of maintaining the confidentiality of all information that study participants share with them.

Interviewers may also need to complete additional institution-mandated research ethics training sessions.

The bulk of the training session is then usually dedicated to understanding and practicing the interview process. The questionnaire should be examined in detail so that all interviewers understand what each question is asking, how to pronounce all the words in each question, how to phrase the reading of each question, and how to present the possible answers for questions that are not open-ended. All paper response forms and/or computer-assisted data entry programs should be closely examined so that every interviewer understands exactly how to record participant responses. Each interviewer should have the opportunity to participate in several mock interviews from start to finish, including the informed consent process. Clear guidelines and lots of practice will help to create skilled and confident interviewers (FIGURE 19-4).

Characteristic	Actions That Demonstrate the Characteristic
Respectful	• Communicates pleasantly and professionally with all study participants and members of the research team • Has practiced interviewing enough to be comfortable with both the script and the interview process • Asks supervisors for assistance when it is needed
Organized	• Begins each scheduled interview session on time • Has all necessary materials on hand prior to the start of each interview session • Maintains meticulous records and completes all files and paperwork promptly
Considerate	• Dresses and grooms appropriately for in-person interviews • Is alert to modifiable conditions that may make interviewees uncomfortable, such as loud background noises or dim lighting • Allows adequate time for participants to respond to each question
Articulate	• Speaks at an appropriate pace and volume • Enunciates clearly • Uses an appropriate tone of voice (and, for in-person interviews, appropriate facial expressions and gestures) • Rereads questions and/or the list of close-ended responses when a participant does not understand the question or acceptable responses
Consistent	• Reads the script exactly as it is written • Probes for answers only when the script indicates that probing is approved • Does not provide explanations for any question unless an explanation is provided in the script or approved in the interviewer handbook
Impartial	• Avoids verbal and nonverbal expressions of approval or disapproval • Does not express personal opinions • Avoids leading interviewees toward a particular answer (for example, by placing special emphasis on particular words in a question or by probing until receiving a particular desired response)
Honest	• Does not fabricate or falsify reports • Records responses to open-ended questions verbatim, without rephrasing, paraphrasing, "correcting," or interpreting them
Careful	• Completes all steps of the interview process in the correct order, as prescribed by the interviewer handbook • Documents informed consent prior to conducting an interview • Does not skip any component of the interview • Completes all response forms correctly

FIGURE 19-4 Characteristics of Well-Trained Interviewers

Primary Studies: Additional Assessments

CHAPTER

20

Surveys and interviews are the most common sources of health data, but other measurements are often important supplements to self-reported information.

20.1 Supplementing Self-Reported Information

Self-reports, such as those made during interviews and the completion of questionnaires, are essential data sources, but they have significant limitations. Respondents may not tell the truth, either because they do not accurately remember the answers or because they want to provide "correct" answers. Also, they may not know some of their health measures, such as their current weight or blood pressure. Laboratory tests and other objective measures can be used to supplement and validate self-reported data and to explore factors that require independent assessment. This information is usually collected in person by a member of the research team. This chapter presents some of these additional types of data.

20.2 Anthropometric Measures

Anthropometry is the measurement of the human body, and *anthropometric measurements* are often important, especially in studies of nutritional status. Some of the most common body measurements are:

147

- Height (stature)
- Weight
- Waist circumference
- Hip circumference
- Mid-upper arm circumference
- Skinfold measurements that estimate the body fat percentage

Standardized methods should be used to take these measurements. Any tools used for the measurements should be carefully calibrated to ensure accuracy and reliability. The individuals taking the measurements should be trained to use all equipment properly and to record results to the appropriate level of precision. They should also ensure privacy for participants while the measurements are taken.

■ 20.3 Vital Signs

Basic vital signs are physiological measurements that can be accurately taken after minimal instruction. These include:

- Temperature
- Blood pressure
- Pulse (heart rate)
- Respiratory rate (breathing frequency)

A thermometer is used to measure body temperature. A manual or electronic sphygmomanometer (a blood pressure cuff) is used to measure systolic and diastolic blood pressure. Resting pulse and respiratory rate do not require any instruments other than timekeeping devices. All assessors should be trained to use the same techniques, and tests of inter-rater reliability should be used to confirm that all assessors get similar or identical results when they measure the same person.

■ 20.4 Clinical Examination

A well-trained clinician can make accurate and reliable assessments of many health states that machines are unable to assess well. A clinician can examine:

- Heart sounds
- Breath sounds and other respiratory functions
- Bowel sounds and the condition of the abdomen
- The range of motion (ROM) and the condition of the joints
- The condition of the skin, hair, and nails
- The health of the eyes, ears, nose, and mouth
- Mental status

- The ability to conduct activities of daily living
- Other signs of health or disease

Sometimes a clinical examination will be part of the data collection process. If so, an assessment form should carefully describe each component of the examination, including the exact procedures to be used and the specific diagnostic criteria for each item on the assessment form, as well as the order in which these elements should be examined.

■ 20.5 Tests of Physiological Function

Tests of physiological function can provide helpful information about health status. For example, spirometry measures lung function, electrocardiography (ECG) measures heart function, electroencephalography (EEG) measures brain function, and audiometry measures hearing acuity.

■ 20.6 Laboratory Analysis of Biological Specimens

Tests of serum, urine, stool, saliva, and/or other biological specimens may be helpful for identifying:

- The risk factors for a disease
- The presence of a disease or markers for a disease
- The characteristics associated with having a disease

Some studies require the collection of new specimens, either as part of routine clinical practice or specifically for the purposes of the research project. If so, a research ethics committee must be assured that the potential physical risks to participants caused by the collection of the sample will be minimized and that the privacy of participants will be protected.

Some studies may be able to make use of existing specimen banks, whether the samples are anonymous or linked to other information about the donor. The use of existing samples also requires ethics committee review and approval. Participants may have a right to the results of the laboratory tests conducted on their own biological specimens, and the protocol should discuss how notification will occur.

■ 20.7 Medical Imaging

Medical imaging techniques are sometimes used to visualize parts of the human body. Examples are radiography (X-rays), magnetic resonance imaging (MRI), computed tomography (CT), and ultrasound. The resulting images may be useful to researchers for purposes of diagnosis and/or for the assessment of responses to therapies.

■ 20.8 Tests of Physical Fitness

A number of different tests can be used to measure physical fitness levels.

- Cardiorespiratory fitness can be assessed using a 1-mile walking test, a 1.5-mile run test, or some other test of aerobic fitness.
- Measures of muscle strength and endurance include timed curl-ups, push-ups, pull-ups, flexed arm hangs, bench presses, leg presses, and grip tests (using a hand-grip dynamometer).
- Flexibility can be measured using a sit-and-reach test (often measured with a flex-ometer) and other activities that stretch the lower back, hamstrings, or other muscle groups.
- Additional tests of fitness may assess agility, balance, coordination, speed, power, and reaction time.

■ 20.9 Environmental Assessment

Both the natural and built environment can have an impact on human health. Exposure to polluted air or water or to toxic substances (such as asbestos, lead, mercury, radon, or pesticides) can compromise health. Access to outdoor recreational areas and the installation of safety equipment, like grab bars in the bathrooms of older adults, can contribute to increased health. Some research projects may benefit from measuring the levels of environmental contaminants or the presence of hazards in the home and/or work environments of research participants. For example, the amount of radon in the lowest floor of a participant's home, the presence of lead in paint chips from the home, and/or the amount of daily precipitation falling at a participant's home location could be linked to a health questionnaire.

■ 20.10 GIS (Geographic Information Systems)

Sometimes a map and/or spatial analysis of important features in the study area would help answer the study question. If so, a *GPS (global positioning system) receiver* can be used to acquire the geographic coordinates (in latitude, longitude, and altitude) for relevant locations, such as the homes of participants, hospitals and other healthcare facilities, roads, schools, houses of worship, grocery stores, recreation facilities, water sources, and industrial sites. The coordinates for public locations can be collected by anyone, but permission from the owners or residents of private land may be needed before entering their property to take a GPS reading. The GPS coordinates for the homes of participants is identifying information; extra care must be taken to protect this data (see Chapter 21).

Primary Studies: Ethical Considerations

> *Researchers have an ethical obligation to minimize the risks that research may pose to participants.*

■ 21.1 Beneficence, Autonomy, and Justice

The three main principles in biomedical research ethics are beneficence, autonomy (sometimes called "respect for persons"), and distributive justice. Each protocol should be carefully inspected to ensure its compliance with these principles. This sort of scrutiny is required by research ethics committees, and, more importantly, researchers need to adhere to the highest standards of professionalism.

Beneficence means that the study should "do good" and is often paired with *nonmaleficence*, which means that the study should "do no harm." To meet the requirement of beneficence, a research proposal must have a high likelihood of benefitting individual participants and/or the communities from which they are drawn. For most studies, the opportunity to contribute to scientific knowledge is considered an adequate benefit to participants, although in some cases more specific individual and community benefits can be offered.

Nonmaleficence requires that steps be taken to minimize potential physical, psychological, financial, social, or other harms to participants, as well as to ensure an acceptable balance between risks and benefits. For example, the principle of doing no harm means that experimental studies must identify ahead of time what events would

Category	Examples of Questions to Ask
Contribution	• Why is the proposed project important? • How will individuals and/or communities benefit from this study?
Compensation	• Will individuals or communities that participate in the study be offered any form of inducement, reimbursement, or compensation? If so, what will be offered, and is it appropriate? Is the offer so high that it could be seen as coercive or so low that the study could be seen as exploitative? • Are the risks of participation minimal? • How will study-related injuries be handled? • Are the risks and benefits balanced?
Consent	• How will potential participants be informed about the study? • How will consent to participate be documented? • Will a test of comprehension be required? • If applicable, how will consent (and possibly assent) be acquired for children and other members of potentially vulnerable populations? • If applicable, will community meetings be held prior to beginning the study?
Confidentiality	• How will the privacy and confidentiality of participants and their personal information be maintained?
Community	• Why is research in the selected population important? • Is the source population appropriate for the goals of the research study? • Will the selection process be fair? • Will the sample size be adequate? • Are potentially vulnerable participants adequately protected? • Has the protocol been adapted to address the cultural expectations of the source population? • If applicable, has the community agreed to participate in this project?
Conflicts of interest	• Who is contributing to the project's finances and/or logistics? • Might potential conflicts of interest inhibit the ability of a researcher to conduct ethical and unbiased research?
Collaborators	• Are all members of the research team adequately trained to conduct ethical research? • What steps will be taken during data collection and analysis to ensure that the protocol and all ethical standards are adhered to by all members of the research team?
Committees	• Which research ethics committee(s) needs to review the project? • If applicable, what community organizations have been consulted about the proposed project?

FIGURE 21-1 **Eight Central Considerations (8 Cs) in Research Ethics**

lead to early termination of the study. Discontinuation might be appropriate when the intervention appears to be dangerous or when it appears to be so beneficial that it would be unethical not to immediately offer the intervention to those in the placebo group. Another way to minimize harm is to provide participants in studies that might cause emotional distress with information about local counseling services.

Autonomy means that participation in research should be completely voluntary. For almost all research projects that involve interaction with individual participants and/or their personally identifiable records, each potential participant must be fully informed about the benefits and burdens of the study, the procedures involved, and the plans for use of the data collected. They must also be given a free choice to participate or not.

Respect for persons is a broader concept that includes, for example:

- Justifying the necessity for and the importance of the research project
- Choosing an appropriate source population
- Using a fair process to sample and recruit participants
- Ensuring an adequate sample size so that the study has adequate statistical power to assess the study objectives
- Making research procedures as minimally invasive as possible
- Maintaining the confidentiality of all shared information

Distributive justice seeks to ensure that the benefits and burdens of research are equitable. For example, if an experimental pharmaceutical therapy proves to be effective and safe, participants in the clinical trial should be guaranteed continued access to the drug after the trial is over.

FIGURE 21-1 highlights some of the many questions that researchers should ask about their own protocols prior to a formal ethics committee review. International health research guidelines, such as those developed by the Council for International Organizations of Medical Sciences (CIOMS), and national research guidelines may identify additional areas of concern that need to be considered as protocols are developed.

■ 21.2 Incentives

Incentives are sometimes offered to research recruits and participants. Researchers need to consider the ethical implications of offering an inducement to potential participants to encourage them to enroll in a study, of offering reimbursement for the costs of participation, or of compensating participants for their efforts.

Research incentives do not have to be monetary. For nearly every study, a benefit to participants is their contribution to scientific knowledge and to the increased understanding of their own health risks and disease conditions—as well as their communities'—that can result from scientific research. For many research projects in the health sciences, this is sufficient reward for participation. At the same time, the principle of nonmaleficence requires that participation in a research project should not be an undue burden to participants. So in some situations reimbursing participants for their travel expenses or compensating them for their time may be appropriate.

To increase the participation rate, researchers may reasonably offer a small gift to all participants or enter all respondents to a questionnaire into a drawing for a more substantial gift that one randomly selected participant will receive. It may also be appropriate to provide free treatment for certain conditions examined by the study, such as iron pills for participants found to have anemia or de-worming medication for participants with intestinal parasites (so long as the relevant health education materials are also provided to participants receiving these treatments). In the case of clinical trials, covering all medical expenses directly related to participation in the study is sometimes appropriate.

However, the desire to reward participants must be balanced with the need for participation in any research project to be voluntary. When an individual feels coerced into participation, the principle of voluntariness is violated. Coercion could include social pressure or requests from authority figures that make it difficult for an individual not to agree to enroll in a study. For example:

- Employees asked by their supervisors to enroll in an occupational health study may fear losing their jobs if they do not agree to participate.
- Patients asked by their own physicians to register for a research study may fear that their medical care will suffer if they do not comply with the request.
- Prisoners may believe that participation in a research study is mandated and/or will yield unspecified rewards.

Coercion can also include generous incentives, such as free medical care and monetary compensation, that could significantly impair the ability of an individual to make an informed decision about the risks as well as the benefits of participation. To minimize the risk of coercion, researchers have to be very transparent about what participants will gain from participation in a research study and what they will not gain.

■ 21.3 Informed Consent Statements

Informed consent statements provide essential information about research projects to potential research participants so that they can make a reasoned decision about whether to enroll in a study. The key components of an informed consent statement are summarized in FIGURE 21-2. The statement must use clear, simple language that the reader is able to understand to describe the study aims, the procedures and expectations of participants, and the benefits and the possible risks of participation. It should emphasize that participation is voluntary and that any participant can withdraw from the study at any time. Informed consent statements should be tailored to the source population, and they may need to address cultural attitudes, beliefs, and traditions.

Content Area	Description
Research	A definition of "research" and a statement that the study involves research
Purpose	An explanation of the purpose and aims of the research process (except in the rare situations in which that interferes with the research goals)
Participants	A description of how and why certain individuals or communities were invited to participate in the research project and an estimate of the total number of individuals who will be recruited
Procedures	A description of the study procedures (including any physical exams, collection of biological samples, randomization or blinding processes, interventions, or other procedures that are part of the study protocol) and the expected duration of the individual participant's involvement in the study
Benefits	A description of benefits to participants and/or to society, including a clear explanation of the compensation to be offered or a clear statement that the participant will receive no direct benefits
Risks	A description of the possible risks, discomforts, and costs associated with participation, a statement that involvement in the project may involve unforeseeable risks, and a description of how study-related injuries will be handled
Confidentiality	A description of the steps that will be taken to maintain confidentiality
Voluntariness	A statement that participation is voluntary and that the participant may withdraw from the study at any time with no penalty, along with an explanation for the process of withdrawing from the study
Contact information	Contact information for the researchers
Signature	Space for the participant's signature

FIGURE 21-2 Content for the Informed Consent Statement

■ 21.4 Informed Consent Process

Although researchers are often more concerned about acquiring a signature from participants than explaining the research process to them, informed consent is intended to be a process, not merely a piece of paper. The principle of autonomy dictates that potential participants in a research study have the right to make their own decisions about whether to participate and that they must be provided with information that will allow them to make informed choices.

The informed consent process consists of the following steps:

- Reading the informed consent statement aloud to a potential participant and/or allowing the individual to read a copy of the statement

- Allowing adequate time for the potential participant to consider whether he or she wants to participate
- Answering any questions
- Only then asking whether the individual wants to participate in the study and is willing to sign an informed consent form

Acquiring a signature is not the end of the process. The lines of communication between researchers and participants must remain open during and after the data collection process. All participants must be given a copy of the informed consent statement that includes contact information so that they can contact the researchers if they have concerns about the study or desire to withdraw.

The researcher should ensure that participants understand the research process and the consent document. A brief test of comprehension may be helpful. For example, recruits for an intervention study may be asked to say in their own words what "randomization" means. A correct answer will demonstrate an understanding that each participant may be assigned to a control group rather than to the active intervention group and that participants do not have a choice in the matter. An incorrect or incomplete answer may require additional explanation of the research process prior to acquisition of a signature on a consent document.

■ 21.5 Informed Consent Documentation

For most studies, the expectation is that each study participant will sign a printed copy of the informed consent statement. This written record provides legal protection for the institution sponsoring the research project because it shows that participants agreed to the terms of the study. For telephone interviews, informed consent documents may be mailed to potential participants, signed, and mailed back to researchers prior to the interview. For computer-based surveys, an electronic signature can be provided.

In some situations, written consent is not appropriate, such as when participants could be harmed by being linked to the study or when the source population has a low literacy rate. When few potential participants are able to read and write, participants might provide a thumbprint or some other mark to indicate consent. Alternatively, when it is inappropriate to ask people who cannot read a document to sign it, oral consent may be preferable. Oral (or verbal) consent must usually be witnessed by an independent third person (someone other than the researcher or the participant), and in some cases a statement of consent is also audio-recorded.

In a limited number of studies, the individual informed consent process may not be required. Some anonymous questionnaires do not require an intense informed consent process if they:

- Cannot be linked to individuals
- Do not ask sensitive questions

- Do not physically examine individuals or collect biological specimens
- Are so short that describing the study would take longer than completing the questionnaire

In these situations, when there are no foreseeable risks to participants, the completion of the survey can sometimes be considered adequate proof of willingness to participate.

Other studies might also not require consent. For example, if researchers will observe groups of individuals in public places, where participants have no reasonable expectation of privacy and will not interact with the researchers, consent is not required.

Different research ethics committees will have different levels of comfort with waiving consent or allowing alternative methods for documenting consent. The relevant committees should be consulted about what they will consider acceptable.

■ 21.6 Confidentiality and Privacy

Privacy is the assurance that individuals have the right to choose what information they reveal about themselves. The right to privacy means that:

- Individuals have the right to refuse to allow their personal information to be shared with researchers.
- Individuals who agree to participate in a study involving face-to-face interviews should have the option of meeting with researchers in a place where no one outside the research team will be able to observe or overhear the interview.

Confidentiality is the protection of personal information provided to researchers. One way to guarantee confidentiality is not to collect any personally identifiable information, such as names, addresses, identification numbers, or other data that can be linked to an individual. This is often an option for cross-sectional surveys, but it is not possible for prospective or longitudinal studies in which baseline data about individuals must be linked to their own follow-up data. When individually identifying information must be collected, many steps throughout the research process can be taken to protect the information.

- All paper records should be stored in a locked file box in a locked room, and all computerized data files should be password-protected.
- Names and other personal identifiers should not be included in data files that contain sensitive personal information. Instead, two separate files should be created, one for identifying information and one for all other data. These should be linked only by a unique study identification number.
- Only essential research personnel should have access to the file containing personally identifying information.

- At some point after the end of the study (and in compliance with the rules of the relevant research ethics committees about how long documentation of informed consent must be stored), individually identifying records should be destroyed.

Researchers asking questions about sensitive issues must decide ahead of time how to handle disclosures. In some situations, guaranteeing confidentiality may not be possible if doing so would violate the law. For example, legal mandates may oblige researchers to alert the police about child abuse, intimate partner violence, or suicidal ideation, or to inform public health authorities about diagnoses of some infections. The decision about how to collect data related to these issues may require consultation with a legal expert and local authorities. Participants in studies of serious genetic diseases should be offered genetic counseling and given the opportunity to decide whether they want to know the results of tests.

A research ethics committee may waive the usual requirement that consent forms include the names of participants if a study will collect information that could cause harm to the participants if their names could be linked to the study. This may include studies of:

- Drug or alcohol abuse
- Sexual practices and preferences
- Psychiatric illnesses
- Immigration status
- Participation in illegal activities
- Genetic disorders

If the study will examine any of these potentially sensitive areas, the ethics committee should be consulted early on in the planning process so that appropriate protocols for handling the information can be developed.

■ 21.7 Cultural Considerations

A protocol must be appropriate to the culture or cultures of the expected study participants. Culturally appropriate recruiting may take different forms. For example, in some cultures, a small gift may be expected as a token of goodwill before an individual is asked to participate in a study. In other parts of the world, this would be considered coercive because it would create a "debt" owed to the researcher. In some cultures, participants may expect a small gift upon completion of the study. In other cultures, such a gesture of appreciation might make volunteers feel that the gift somehow devalues their donation to science. Participants from some cultures expect to share tea or a light meal with researchers before any questions are asked. People from other cultures may expect that all health research will be conducted in a clinical setting. In some parts of the world, prospective participants might need to know that community leaders, such as government officials, religious leaders, or tribal leaders, have approved of the project and are monitoring it. In other cultures, the association of authorities with a research project may raise concerns about voluntariness, confidentiality, and/or the potential misuse of data.

The informed consent process may also need to be adapted to local custom. Although individual participants are always required to provide consent for their own participation, potential participants may need time to consult with their spouses, parents, or other family members prior to giving consent. For some community-based studies, a meeting of the whole community should be held so that everyone is confident that they are all hearing the same story from the researchers. It may be helpful to have a local advisory board serve as the intermediaries between the community and the research team. The informed consent statement and study materials may need to be available in multiple languages.

The survey instruments and data collection process must also be culturally appropriate, and researchers must be trained in culturally respectful interview techniques. Topics that are openly discussed in one culture may be sensitive in another. Tests that are only mildly uncomfortable in one culture may be extremely distressing in another. For example, although people in some cultures are sensitive about the measurement of body weight, other cultures may not care about weight but may be uncomfortable with the measurement of height. There may be formal or informal restrictions on who can conduct an interview or a physical examination. Female participants may be unwilling to be examined by a male, or older participants may be uncomfortable being interviewed by a much younger person. Participants may expect to be alone with just a researcher, but in other cases participants will expect to have a family member present for the entire process.

If the research team does not include members of the target population, it is important to work with representatives of the source community when developing and revising the protocol. Additionally, some research ethics committees require a cultural expert to examine the protocol as part of the review process.

■ 21.8 Vulnerable Populations

Vulnerable populations are discussed in Chapter 16. In addition to defending why a particular research project must focus on a potentially vulnerable population, extra care must be taken to ensure that:

- The selection process is fair.
- Potential participants are assured that participation is voluntary.
- Participants (and/or their legal representatives) are fully informed about the possible benefits and risks of the study as well as about the expectations of participants.

Although most members of vulnerable populations can make their own choices about whether to participate in a research project, children and some adults with cognitive impairments may not be considered competent to make an informed decision. In this situation, a legally approved guardian is allowed to grant consent on behalf of the study participant. Whenever possible, in addition to having the legal representative's *consent*, potential participants should *assent* to their own participation.

■ 21.9 Ethics Training and Certification

Research ethics committees usually require everyone who will be in direct contact with research participants and/or their personal data to complete formal research ethics training. Many institutions offer their own courses, either in-person or online, and several funding agencies and nonprofit organizations also offer training that is available to anyone. After completing modules on various aspects of research ethics and passing an exam, a certificate of completion (usually valid for one to three years) is issued, affirming that the investigator has been trained in ethics. Copies of these certificates should be saved because research ethics committees often require proof of ethics training for all members of the research team.

Ethical Review and Approval

> *Research ethics committees protect study participants, researchers, and host institutions by carefully reviewing research protocols prior to their implementation.*

■ 22.1 Ethics Committee Responsibilities

The three primary goals of *research ethics committees* (RECs), often called *Institutional Review Boards* (IRBs) in the United States, are to:

- Protect the "human subjects" who will participate in observational or experimental studies or whose personal information will be examined by researchers. (Separate animal care and use committees oversee research with animals.)
- Legally protect the researcher's institution from the liability that could occur as a result of research activities.
- Protect researchers by preventing them from engaging in activities that could cause harm.

The major functions of ethics review boards are to:

- Review new and revised research protocols
- Approve or disapprove of those protocols
- Ensure that informed consent is documented (if required)
- Conduct continuing review of long-term research projects

■ 22.2 Warning: Ethics Review Takes Time

Research ethics committees are usually composed of at least five members, preferably from diverse backgrounds, including scientists and nonscientists. Each member reviews the proposal and then meets with the others to discuss it and to decide about whether it meets the ethical requirements of the institution. An outside scientific expert and/or community representative may also be consulted about the research plan. As a result, even the most efficient ethics review committees, when reviewing even the simplest proposals, may need a month or longer to issue an exemption or an approval or to make a request for a revision to be made to the protocol, which must then be reconsidered by the committee before final approval. For complicated proposals, the review may take several months. Examples are studies involving:

- Invasive procedures
- Sensitive questions
- Potentially harmful interventions
- Deception about the study aims
- Waiver of written informed consent
- Multiple sites
- International research teams

A research time line should assume a lengthy review period. The application should therefore be submitted to the ethics committee as soon as possible in the planning process.

■ 22.3 Application Materials

Some research ethics committees ask applicants to provide a narrative research statement that addresses a list of possible ethical concerns. Others require the completion of dozens of pages of forms that require answers to a long series of questions about the project (even though most questions require an answer of only "no" or "not applicable"). FIGURE 22-1 summarizes the questions that research ethics committees commonly examine during the review process. A research protocol or narrative statement about a planned project should address each of these points and any others required by the committees evaluating the proposal.

Proposals for the analysis of existing data may be significantly shorter than proposals for new data collection, but both primary and secondary analysis proposals need to:

- Describe the expected study participants
- Discuss the risks and benefits of the study
- Explain how confidentiality will be ensured

Category	Considerations
Participants	• What is the anticipated composition and size of the study population? • How will participants be recruited? Does the recruitment method raise any concerns about coercion? • What are the inclusion and exclusion criteria? Are they reasonable? • Is the source population appropriate for the study question? • Are potentially vulnerable subjects protected, if applicable?
Risks and benefits	• Why is the study important and necessary? How will the proposed study benefit participants and/or their communities? • How will data be collected? Will existing data, documents, records, or specimens be used? Will individuals or groups be examined using surveys, interviews, focus groups, oral histories, program evaluations, or other methods? Will data be audio or video recorded? Will noninvasive clinical measures be taken? Will participants be asked to engage in exercise or tests of endurance, strength, or flexibility? What machines will be used to collect data, and will collection involve radiation exposure? Will blood, hair, nail clippings, sweat, saliva, sputum, skin cells, or other biological specimens be collected noninvasively? Will drugs or devices be tested? • What are the potential physical, psychological, financial, or other risks to participants? • Are the risks minimal (or at least minimized)? • Are the risks reasonable compared to the anticipated benefits?
Informed consent	• Does the informed consent statement adhere to institutional guidelines? • How will informed consent be sought? • How will informed consent be documented? • Is any modification to the usual methods of documenting informed consent being requested? Is the request reasonable? (For example, are parents being asked to provide consent for their children, and are the children being asked to assent to participation? Or is a waiver of a signed consent form being requested because the source population has a low literacy rate? Or is a request being made to have no documentation of consent because the existence of a form linking an individual to the study could harm the participant?)
Privacy and confidentiality	• How will privacy and confidentiality be maintained? • What are the plans for the protection of computerized and noncomputerized data?
Safety monitoring	• Does the informed consent statement clearly state how research participants can contact the research team and/or the ethics review board if they have concerns? • What constitutes an adverse event? How will such events be handled?

FIGURE 22-1 Examples of Information Requested and Examined by Ethics Review Committees

Category	Considerations
Conflicts of interest	• How is the project being funded? • Do any financial or personal conflicts of interest need to be disclosed and/or addressed?
Researcher training	• Are the investigators prepared to conduct ethical research?
Documentation	• Are copies of all recruitment materials (if any) attached? • Are copies of the questionnaire and/or other assessment tools attached? • Is a copy of the informed consent statement attached? • Are copies of letters of approval from study sites and/or other ethics review committees attached, if applicable? • Is a copy of the grant proposal attached, if applicable? • Are copies of research ethics training certificates for all members of the research team attached?

FIGURE 22-1 (continued)

- Disclose potential conflicts of interest
- Provide proof of ethics training
- Supply all relevant documentation

For primary studies, the documentation may include a copy of the informed consent statement, the questionnaire, and recruiting materials. For secondary analyses, the application must include evidence that the data are in the public domain or that appropriate individuals or organizations have granted the researcher permission to analyze the data.

■ 22.4 Review Process

Once all application materials have been submitted to a research ethics committee, there are three possible next steps: (1) exemption, (2) expedited review, and (3) full review. The ethics review board decides which action is appropriate.

Exemption from review may be granted—but does not have to be granted—when the research involves the analysis of existing records or existing biological specimens that cannot be linked to individuals.

An exemption can also be granted for data collected as part of normal practice that is not intended to contribute to generalizable knowledge. It is important to make a distinction between routine practice activities and intentional research activities. Practice activities include teachers assessing their students' knowledge of class material, clinicians examining their patients, community health organizations initiating monitoring and evaluation projects, and public health officials collecting surveillance data and conducting outbreak investigations. None of these activities requires review by a research ethics committee; all are considered to be within the accepted scope of practice. However, ethics review is required if these practitioners or organizations choose to engage in research activities.

- An educator plans to have students take special pre- and post-tests to assess a new pedagogical approach and hopes to publish the results in a teaching journal.
- A clinician reviews patient records so that they can be presented as a case series at a professional conference.
- The results of a survey of clients of a community organization might later be published in a professional journal.

In such situations, an exemption might be appropriate, but the decision is up to the committee, not the researcher.

An *expedited review* may be possible when a minor change to a previously approved protocol is requested. Sometime expedited review is also possible for new studies in which the risk to participants is no greater than what is encountered in ordinary daily life (or, in the case of clinical work, during routine examinations). Expedited review may allow the chair of the ethics committee to approve the proposal without a full meeting of the committee. However, all members must be notified of the decision and given an opportunity to express concerns.

Full review of the research proposal is usually required when data will be collected through interaction with individuals, an intervention will be tested in individuals or a community, or identifiable private information will be collected. The ethics review committee has the right to approve the proposal or to deny approval. If a protocol is not satisfactory at initial review, the committee usually informs the investigators of changes to the protocol that the committee feels will make the proposal acceptable. Some requests may be easy to accommodate, and researchers should simply comply with them. At other times, the requested changes would significantly alter the nature of the project or would be unfeasible given the intended study population. In this situation, the researchers need to present their concerns to the ethics review committee and to try to work with them to find an acceptable resolution. However, the committee does not have to acquiesce to the desires of the researchers. The ethics review board has the right (and sometimes the duty) to deny approval to any protocol that does not meet its standards. Furthermore, the board can demand proof that certain standards (for example, standards for data storage or investigator training) are met prior to approving the protocol.

■ 22.5 Review by Multiple Committees

Multiple research ethics committees may be required to review studies that involve researchers from multiple institutions and/or participants from multiple countries or multiple study sites. Additionally, funding agencies may require review by their own ethics boards. For example, a student planning on conducting thesis research in an-other country must have the research protocol reviewed by, at minimum, two ethics boards: one from his or her own university and one from an ethics committee in the study country (often a local university or a teaching hospital).

At least three issues must be resolved prior to submission of a research proposal to multiple committees: the application documents that will be required, the wording of the informed consent statement, and the order of review.

First, each review board must be consulted about the application materials it wants to receive. Sometimes submitting the same paperwork to all committees is possible. More likely, each board will require its own unique application materials, perhaps in addi-tion to copies of all documents submitted to other ethics committees. The researchers have the responsibility to ensure that each application packet describes the study ob-jectives and protocol in the same way.

Second, many institutions have their own preferred wording for informed con-sent statements. The informed consent statement is seen as a legal document, and in-stitutions want to be sure that the wording protects them. However, the preferred wording may differ for each participating institution. A resolution about how to merge consent statement requirements—while making sure that the study participants will understand the language—must be reached.

Third, the order of review must be established. Sometimes all the committees in-dependently review the proposal at the same time. Other times the reviews are con-ducted "domino" style, with the proposal being independently reviewed and approved by one committee, then passed to the next committee, and so on. Committees com-monly stipulate that approval by their institution will be contingent on approval from all other participating institutions, even when they review concurrently. If a modifica-tion of the protocol or informed consent document is mandated by one committee, then all other committees must re-review the proposal. A significant amount of extra time for ethics review should be built into the project time line when multiple research ethics committees will be involved.

■ 22.6 Ongoing Review

Studies that can be completed within one year may not require further contact with the research ethics committee after initial approval. Usually, however, the researcher is required to provide updates to the committee for the duration of the project. Routine reports about the number of participants recruited may be required. All adverse events must be immediately reported to the ethics review board. Any changes to the informed consent statement, the questionnaire, recruiting materials, or other study documents must receive prior approval. In addition, all ongoing research protocols must be re-reviewed annually (or more often, at the discretion of the ethics review committee) until the completion of data collection or, in some cases, until the completion of data analysis. The progress report for re-review may need to include (depending on institutional requirements):

- Current versions of the protocol, informed consent statement, questionnaire, and other study documents
- A report on the number of participants enrolled in the study, including basic demographic information about them
- A report of any adverse events or complaints
- A list of any amendments to the protocol or study materials that are being requested
- A summary of findings (which are especially important for experimental studies that might need to be stopped early if the intervention appears to be harmful or very beneficial)

■ 22.7 Conflicts of Interest

Most ethics review committees and an increasing number of journals require researchers to disclose potential conflicts of interest related to the study. A potential *conflict of interest* is mostly likely to occur when:

- A new product is being tested, such as a new medication or medical device, and one or more members of the research team earns a salary (or a consulting fee or an honorarium) from or holds equity interests (like stocks or ownership) in the company that produced, developed, or will market the product.
- Intellectual property rights (such as the ownership of a patent or copyright) may result in earnings for one or more researchers.

When a financial or other interest could bias the design, conduct, or reporting of the study—or could merely appear to have the possibility of biasing the study—the potential conflict of interest must be disclosed. The disclosure of a potential conflict of interest is not a confession that bias has occurred or will occur. It is, however, an important assurance of transparency. Most universities and other institutions involved in scientific research have policies about what constitutes a conflict of interest and about when and how potential conflicts need to be disclosed.

■ 22.8 Is Ethics Review Required?

Ethics review is required for almost every proposal that will involve human subjects, whether those people will be directly contacted by the research team (in person, by telephone, by mail, by Internet, or via any other method) or their existing personal information will be analyzed. A small subset of projects might be exempted from review, but the decision to exempt a project from review can be made only by the relevant committees. Researchers are not allowed simply to declare that their projects do not need to be reviewed.

Many incentives are in place to encourage participation in the formal review process. First, institutional approval provides a degree of legal protection to the researcher. An approval letter is evidence that the research plan was carefully considered and deemed reasonably safe by a committee of experts prior to the initiation of data collection and analysis. Another incentive is that some granting agencies will not release funds until a research plan has been approved by a research ethics committee. Finally, an increasing number of journals are requiring that authors provide details about which research ethics committee(s) reviewed the project (even if it was subsequently exempted from review). Some are even requiring copies of the official approval letters. Therefore, researchers must take the time to undergo a formal review prior to collecting any data or analyzing any data files. Research protocols cannot be retroactively approved.

Secondary Studies: Existing Data Sets

Some health research studies analyze existing clinical records, survey data, or population data rather than collecting new information from study participants.

■ 23.1 Overview of Secondary Analysis

In some situations, data collection means acquiring existing data sets for secondary analysis. These data files may be publicly available individual-level or population-level data, privately held survey data, or filed clinical records. Whatever the data source, what makes a project a *secondary analysis* is that the researcher conducting the statistical analysis has not had (and does not have) any contact with the individuals whose data are being examined.

A researcher conducting a secondary analysis contributes to scientific knowledge by analyzing and interpreting accumulated data that might otherwise remain untapped. Sometimes a researcher can download an entire data set from an Internet website or have it sent by e-mail. Such files often contain already cleaned data that are ready to analyze within minutes of receipt. At other times, the data are available only as paper or electronic records from which the relevant information must be extracted and entered into a computer database prior to analysis.

■ 23.2 Publicly Available Data Sets

A growing number of governmental agencies (and sometimes research teams supported by federal funds and private organizations) make their data sets available to the public or routinely make data available to researchers upon request. These organizations are experts at collecting data but often do not have the resources to conduct a thorough statistical analysis of an entire data set before it becomes relatively obsolete. Sharing data is therefore a cost-efficient way to extract as much information as possible out of data sets, especially when the data were expensive to collect. For example, the U.S. Centers for Disease Control and Prevention (CDC) provides, on its website, data from several nationwide cross-sectional studies, including the National Health and Nutrition Examination Survey (NHANES), the National Health Interview Survey (NHIS), and the Behavioral Risk Factor Surveillance System (BRFSS). Statistics Canada provides access to data sets such as the Canadian Community Health Survey (CCHS) via the Research Data Centres Program. The United Kingdom's Medical Research Council has a Data Support Service to link researchers to available population health data. Additional data sets are available from United Nations agencies like the World Health Organization and from various national governments.

Researchers may be able to download an entire data set immediately and at no cost directly from the website of the sponsoring organization. Sometimes there is a screening process. The researcher is required to submit a request form, which must be approved by an oversight body before the requestor can be provided with a copy of the data by e-mail or via a link to a password-protected download site. Although these data files are often provided at no cost to the researcher, sometimes they must be purchased, and access to some data files is limited to citizens or residents of the country in which the data were collected.

A researcher conducting secondary analysis needs to understand all the methods that were used for data collection and the contents of the data file. So, in addition to downloading the data files, the researcher should download and read all supporting documents, such as the project overview, protocol, or handbook; the questionnaire; the codebook; and any published articles that describe the origins of the data set.

Investigators who make their data available to the public often do not expect to be coauthors on papers written by independent analysts. However, they may expect their contributions to be recognized and/or the sources of funding and technical support to be acknowledged. The supporting documents should state the expectations; if they do not, the researcher should ask a contact person for clarification. Also, sometimes the analysis requires assistance from the individuals involved in designing the study and/or collecting and processing the data. If so, those individuals may qualify for coauthorship even if the supporting documentation does not say that this is necessary, and those individuals should be asked about their expectations.

There are some major limitations to using already available data. One is that the analyst is limited to exploring only the topics included in the original survey. A related concern is that the analyst has to trust that the data were collected using valid and standardized methods and that the supporting documentation accurately describes the actual procedures used for data collection. Another challenge is that finding someone who can answer questions about the procedures used might be difficult. Some download websites do not list the name of a contact person, and some of the listed contacts may not have been integrally involved in the study design and data collection process. A final issue is the risk of duplicating the analysis that someone else has done or is doing. A literature search may uncover related works that have been published or are in press, but it will not identify analysis in progress or papers under review by a journal. The contact person for the data set may not know whether other researchers are conducting an analysis of the data or what topics other researchers are focusing on.

Despite its difficulties, secondary analysis is often an excellent option for researchers with strong statistical skills but limited time and/or data collection resources.

■ 23.3 Private Data Sets

Individual researchers and small research teams may have data available that have not yet been analyzed. Sometimes the researchers have computerized data files that have not yet been fully explored. Sometimes paper records have been set aside because they are not a current priority of the research team. Or the original researcher or research team may have published the results of some portion of the data set, but left unanalyzed some of the other potentially significant, interesting, and novel aspects of the data. In this situation, the original researcher may be open to a new researcher taking the lead on analyzing that portion of the data set and writing up the results for possible publication.

A request for access to a private data set is most likely to be granted when the new researcher has some connection to the original researcher. Students are most likely to have success asking their professors for data sets to analyze. Alternatively, if students are interested in the work of a research group at another university or hospital, they may ask their professors to reach out to colleagues at the other institution.

When privately held data are shared with a new investigator, the original researchers usually expect to be coauthors on any resulting publication. The roles and responsibilities of each party should be agreed on as early as possible.

■ 23.4 Clinical Records

Clinical records are a common source of data for case series. Individuals working in clinical settings commonly have access to patient records for research purposes, provided that the research project receives all required approvals and will not violate any law or policy, such as the Health Insurance Portability and Accountability Act (HIPAA) Privacy Rule that must be adhered to in the United States.

Sometimes the relevant information can be extracted from an electronic database. When electronic records are not available, a data extraction form can be created and used to extract the relevant information from each file. The extracted information can be entered directly into a computer database or recorded on paper for later data entry. When possible, the data files should not contain any individually identifying information.

A major limitation of using existing clinical records is that patient records are often incomplete. Researchers cannot assume that missing information is the same as a no. For example, they cannot assume that the absence of information about a symptom means that the patient did not experience the symptom. The patient might have had the symptom but failed to mention it to the clinician. Perhaps the clinician did not specifically ask whether the symptom was occurring. Maybe the patient did mention the symptom but the clinician did not record it, perhaps because the symptom did not seem especially relevant. Similarly, even if a patient's records at one clinical site do not mention that he or she is taking a particular drug, the patient might have been prescribed the medication by a clinician at some other site. When data must be collected in a particular way to be useful to the researcher, a primary study design may be necessary.

■ 23.5 Ethics Committee Review

Additional approval by an ethics committee at the institution where the secondary analysis will be conducted is usually not required if several conditions are met:

- The data to be analyzed are publicly available.
- The data set contains no individually identifying information.
- The data were collected following approval by a federal government or some other widely recognized and reasonably trusted entity.

If the data come from a private source, then, prior to even looking at the data set, the analyst must obtain clearance from his or her own institution and perhaps also from the institution that houses the data. Use of hospital records for research purposes always requires review by a research ethics committee.

Researchers with questions about whether their project requires review should consult the appropriate ethics committees. It is better to err on the side of submitting a perhaps unnecessary proposal than to erroneously presume that a project is exempt from review without confirming the validity of this assumption. Chapter 22 provides information about the ethics review process.

Tertiary Studies: Systematic Reviews and Meta-Analyses

A systematic review is the careful compilation and summary of all publications relevant to a particular research topic. A meta-analysis creates a summary statistic for the results of systematically identified articles.

■ 24.1 Overview of the Systematic Review Process

As noted in the introduction to reviews of the literature in Chapter 7, the *systematic review* process requires the

- Identification of an appropriately narrow study question.
- Selection of a well-defined search strategy.
- Screening of *all* potentially relevant articles to determine whether they meet the predefined eligibility criteria.
- Extraction of relevant information from all eligible articles.
- Summary of the findings of these articles.

FIGURE 24-1 summarizes the systematic review process. In some situations it is appropriate to create a summary statistic by pooling data from the included studies, a process called "meta-analysis," but this is not required.

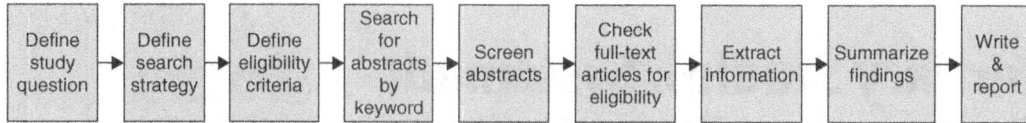

FIGURE 24-1 Systematic Review Process

■ 24.2 Search Strategy

After identifying a well-defined study question, the next critical step in a systematic review or meta-analysis is to select appropriate search terms and search limiters. For example, a systematic review might require included articles to:

- Be indexed in MEDLINE with certain specified MeSH terms
- Be written in English
- Be published in or after 1995
- Use a case-control or cohort study design
- Have a minimum sample size of 20 humans

Or a systematic review might involve searching two or more databases with the same set of keywords, allowing publications in any language (assuming that coauthors and friends can assist with translation) and in any publication year, but restricting eligible articles to randomized controlled trials.

Or a systematic review might involve looking up every article cited in an included article to try to fully capture the entire published literature on the topic (a process sometimes called "snowballing"). The goal is a complete, unbiased list of related articles.

To check the appropriateness of search terms, identify a handful of articles known to be relevant to the study question. Then determine whether the search terms capture all of these articles. If the search misses one or more of the reference pieces, then the search strategy needs to be modified. However, this process must not be used to exclude disliked articles, which would cause the inclusion bias that systematic reviews seek to minimize.

Once a *system* for identifying eligible articles is in place, abstract databases are *systematically* searched for articles that meet all the inclusion criteria. If the topic is appropriately narrow, then keyword searches and limiting factors can often reduce the number of abstracts and/or articles that must be screened for eligibility to a reasonable number, often less than 100 articles. Most systematic reviews end up with about 10 to 25 included articles after screening, although some have many more than that. The full text of each of these screened articles must be read to determine final eligibility. Ideally, each article should be assessed by two independent reviewers. FIGURE 24-2 summarizes this process. The count of articles at each step—identification, screening, checks of eligibility, and inclusion in the manuscript—should be included in the research report.

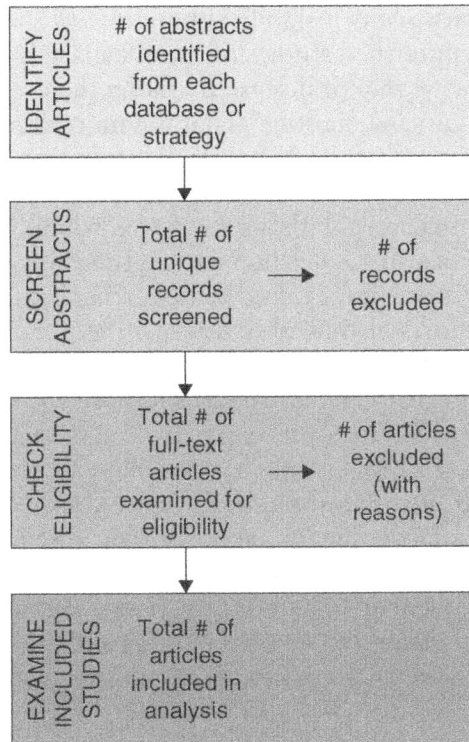

FIGURE 24-2 Systematic Search Strategy and Counts to Report

■ 24.3 Data Extraction

Once all eligible articles are identified, the content of these articles is extracted into *data extraction tables* that list descriptive characteristics like:

- The study location
- The study years
- The study design
- The study population and sample size
- The key findings of interest
- The strengths and limitations of the study

A data extraction table allows for easy compilation and comparison of observations relevant to the study question.

When interpreting the results of a systematic review, studies that find no statistically significant results for an item of interest are just as valuable as those that find a significant association. The researcher should record and report both statistically significant findings ($p < 0.05$) and statistically insignificant findings ($p \geq 0.05$). A report may state, for example, "Five of 40 published studies of the association between exposure A and disease B found an increased rate of disease B among those exposed to A, and the remaining 35 studies found no association." That is a more accurate depiction of the literature than if the report merely says, "Five studies found an increased risk of disease B in those exposed to A." The latter statement incorrectly implies a consensus that exposure A is significantly associated with disease B. One of the primary contributions of systematic reviews to the health science literature is the ability to identify areas of consensus *and* areas of disagreement that need to be further examined.

Systematic review reports also need to address the possible influence of publication bias on the findings. *Publication bias* occurs when articles with statistically significant results are more likely to be published that those with null results. If 10 studies look at the association between the same exposure and the same disease, the one study that finds the exposure to be risky is much more likely to be published than the nine null result studies. Even if the other nine studies are published, they are likely to highlight some other statistically significant aspect of their research and to downplay the lack of a positive or negative association between that exposure and disease. Proving that publication bias has occurred may not be possible, but the presence of consensus should be conservatively interpreted when only a limited number of studies have been published on a topic or the results are mixed.

■ 24.4 Meta-Analysis

A *meta-analysis* pools the results of several studies identified during a systematic review to create one summary statistic. Only similar statistics from similar studies can be pooled. For example, a summary estimate of efficacy can be estimated from several high-quality randomized controlled trials with the same active intervention, the same type of control, and similar population groups. However, the results from studies that use different study designs or dissimilar population groups should not be pooled. Pooling several unadjusted (crude) odds ratios may be appropriate, but pooling a mix of crude odds ratios and age-adjusted odds ratios is usually not.

Before pooling the data, the researcher must show that the results of the studies are comparable. Homogeneous (similar) studies can be combined into a summary statistic, but a great deal of caution should be used if the studies are heterogeneous (dissimilar). The amount of variability in the measure between studies can be examined using a Q-statistic for homogeneity or another appropriate statistic.

If a summary (pooled) statistic appears to be appropriate given the variability among the studies, the next step is to select a model that will be used for creating a pooled estimate of the *effect size*, which is the estimate of a measure like a summary odds ratio, rate ratio, efficacy, correlation coefficient, or difference in means. There are two main choices: a fixed effects model or a random effects model.

- A *fixed effects model* can be used to create a pooled estimate (such as a Mantel-Haenszel adjusted odds ratio) when the studies are fairly homogenous.
- A *random effects model* is required when the tests of heterogeneity show that the included studies are dissimilar.

The point estimate for the summary measure will be similar for both model types. However, a random effects model will result in a wider 95% confidence interval for the summary statistic because the random effects model will adjust for the variability between the included studies.

Once a model is selected, a specialized computer software program can be used to estimate the value of the pooled statistic and its confidence interval. The contribution of each study to the pooled estimate is usually weighted based on the sample size of the included studies, although other approaches to weighting can be used. Step-by-step guides to meta-analysis techniques are available from The Cochrane Collaboration and other resource groups.

The contributing studies and the summary measure are often displayed using a *forest plot* (FIGURE 24-3). A forest plot usually has:

- A horizontal axis showing effect size.
- A vertical line showing the effect size that indicates no effect (such as an odds ratio of 1).
- A row for information from each included study that uses a square or other marker to indicate the point estimate for the effect size and uses a horizontal line to show the 95% confidence interval.
- Markers for the point estimate in varying sizes that show how each study was weighted in the meta-analysis. Small markers usually indicate studies with small sample sizes, and large markers usually indicate studies with large sample sizes.
- A representation of the summary measure, often shown using a diamond shape.

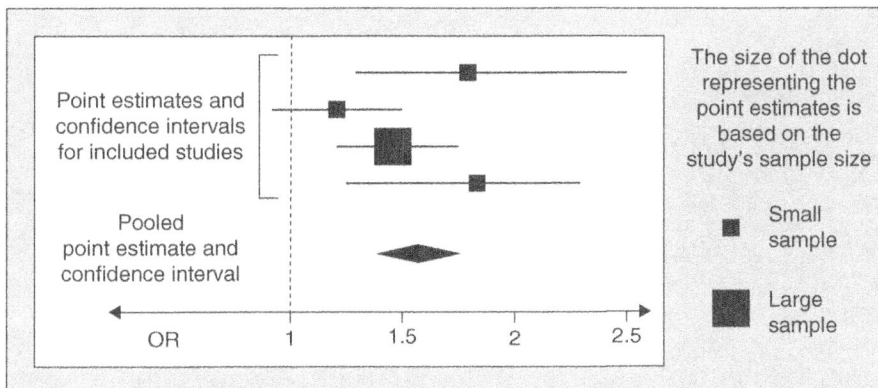

FIGURE 24-3 Example of a Forest Plot

There are two main threats to the validity of a meta-analysis: poor quality of included studies and publication bias. The selection criteria used during the systematic review process can eliminate any studies of questionable validity.

The possibility of publication bias—the preferential publication of studies that report a statistically significant and/or favorable outcome—can be examined using a *funnel plot*. A point for each included study is graphed on a funnel plot that shows effect size on the *x*-axis and sample size on the *y*-axis (FIGURE 24-4). If no publication bias has occurred, the points for the included studies will form a cone shape. If publication bias has reduced the number of publications with statistically insignificant results, a part of the cone will be missing. In that situation, the pooled estimate is likely to have overestimated the true effect size.

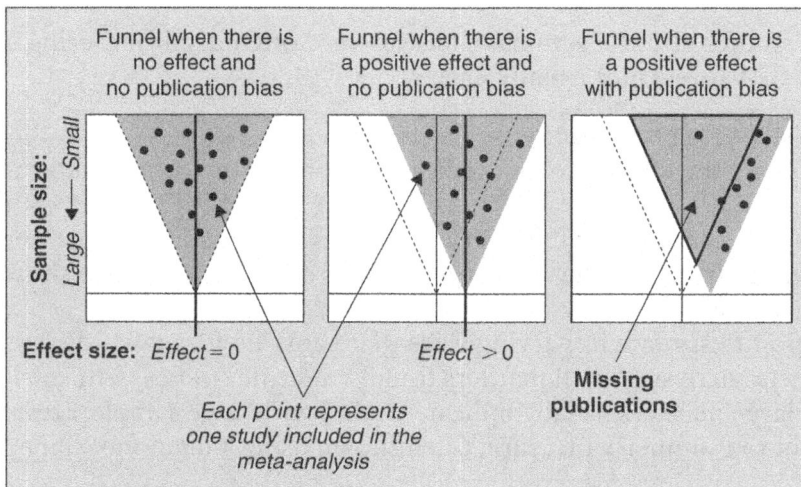

FIGURE 24-4 **Example of a Funnel Plot**

Analyzing Data

Identify study question		Select study approach		Design study & collect data		Analyze data		Report findings

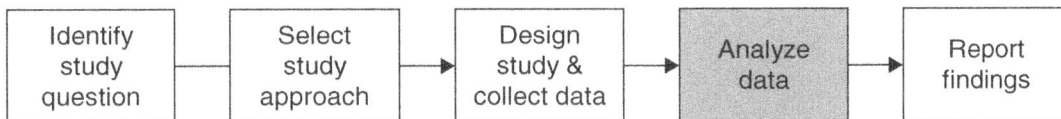

The fourth step in the research process is to compile and analyze the data that were collected during step 3. Most research projects require only the use of descriptive and perhaps some comparative statistics.

- Data management
- Descriptive statistics
- Comparative statistics
- Advanced health statistics

Data Management

> *Data management refers to the entire process of record keeping, whether track-ing articles considered for eligibility in a systematic review, extracting data from patient charts for a case series, entering the responses to a cross-sectional or case-control survey, or recording all the results of clinical assessment conducted dur-ing a longitudinal cohort or experimental study. After data are entered, the files need to be cleaned and perhaps recoded before beginning statistical analysis.*

25.1 Codebooks

Prior to beginning data entry, it is useful to create a *codebook* that describes each vari-able and specifies how the collected information will be entered into a computer data-base (FIGURE 25-1). For quantitative surveys, numeric or alphabetical codes can be assigned to the options for close-ended answers provided on the questionnaire. For open-ended questions and qualitative surveys, a codebook is even more essential because it provides clear instructions for how to code and enter free-response comments.

In addition to providing specific information about how each piece of information should be entered into the computer file, the codebook should specify:

- The name of each variable (which usually employs only capital letters or a com-bination of capital letters and numbers, and avoids starting with a symbol, such as an underscore)
- The wording of the question that was asked
- The variable type
- The options listed on the survey as possible answers to the question

Question Number	Variable Name	Question	Variable Type	Variable Length	Codes
1	INTDATE	{Date of interview}	date	8	• Enter as DD-MM-YYYY
2	AGE	What is your age in years?	numeric	3	• Enter number • *Missing = 999*
3	SEX	What is your sex?	text	1	• Male = M • Female = F • Missing = {*leave blank*}
4	WORK	Which of the following categories best describes your work status?	text	10	• Working full time = FULLTIME • Working part time = PARTTIME • Unemployed but want to work = UNEMP • Retired = RETIRED • Student = STUDENT • Homemaker = HOME • Other = OTHER → *If OTHER go to 4b, otherwise skip to 5*
4b	WORK_OTHER	Other occupational description	text	50	• {Enter text as reported by respondent; only enter for those for whom WORK = OTHER.}
5	STUDENT	Are you currently enrolled in school?	text	1	• Yes = Y • No = N • *Don't know /Missing / Refused = D*

FIGURE 25-1 Example of Codebook Entries

- The way answers should be entered into the computer database
- What to do with missing answers

The codebook is also the place to describe how anticipated data problems will be handled. For example, what should be done if a respondent selects two answers from a multiple choice list when the instructions said to select only one? What should be done if the same person accidentally turns in two copies of the completed survey form? What if the handwriting on a form is illegible or the data entry person is not absolutely certain about what the words say or which box was checked? If unanticipated quandaries arise, the codebook should be amended to state how the situation was addressed.

Question Number	Variable Name	Question	Variable Type	Variable Length	Codes
6	ALC	How often do you drink alcohol?	numeric	1	• Never = 0 • Less than 1 time a month = 1 • About 1 time a month = 2 • About 2 times a month = 3 • About 1 time a week = 4 • About 2–3 times a week = 5 • About 4–5 times a week = 6 • Every day or almost every day = 7 • *Don't know = 8* • *Refused/missing = 9*
7	STD_EVER	Has a doctor ever told you that you had a sexually transmitted disease?	numeric	1	• Yes = 1 • No = 0 • *Don't know = 7* • *Refused to answer = 8* • *Missing = 9*

FIGURE 25-1 (continued)

The codebook will also specify for each variable whether missing answers should be left blank in the database, indicated with a numeric code (such as entering a 9 if the expected entry code is 0 or 1 for a dichotomous variable), or marked with the word "MISSING." The statistical analysis process may need adjustment based on what the codebook says about how missing data were handled. For example, if missing information about age is entered as 999, those entries will need to be removed prior to analysis or else the mean age will end up artificially high and the standard deviation will be very large.

■ 25.2 Data Entry

Data are usually entered into a *database* program (like Microsoft Access). One of the benefits of these programs is that they can be designed to be visually appealing and to include preapproved responses to questions and automatic skips between questions. This ensures the consistency of entries and the completeness of the file.

An alternative option is to enter the data directly into a *spreadsheet* program (like Microsoft Excel). Variable names should be entered in the first row, with one variable per column. Each individual's data should be in a new row. The advantage of this data entry approach is that it does not require creating a data entry form, defining fields and variable names, and doing other coding and testing of the data entry system. The disadvantage is that it is easy to input inconsistent codes, which makes cleaning the data much more difficult, or to accidentally enter new data over an existing row of data.

Both database and spreadsheet files can be uploaded into standard statistical software programs for analysis.

It may be worth doing double-entry of at least some of the completed survey forms (often a minimum of 10% of them) to check the accuracy of data entry. *Double-entry* consists of two individuals entering the same data (or the same person entering the data twice) into two different computer files, then comparing the records in the two files for agreement. Special software programs (such as the Data Compare utility that is part of the U.S. CDC's free Epi Info program) allow the individual records stored in two files to be linked by a unique ID number or other variable and compared. These programs usually provide statistics about the agreement level. If the agreement is not extremely high, then it means that the double-entry and comparison of all records is probably required to ensure the accuracy of the final data file.

The file comparison programs usually facilitate the creation of a clean final data file. They identify disputed entries and allow the researcher to select the best response for the final clean data file after consulting the original survey forms. For example, suppose one of the two database files indicates that a participant was 32 years old, and the other says that the participant was 42 years old. The original form completed by the participant may indicate that the true age is 42, and 42 can be selected as the correct entry for the cleaned file.

■ 25.3 Data Cleaning

Data cleaning is the process of correcting any typographical or other errors in data files. FIGURE 25-2 shows how errors such as extra spaces, typos, and the use of lower-case instead of capital letters can be fixed so that the responses all adhere to the codebook. When paper-based data collection methods are used, fixing incorrect entries sometimes requires looking up the original survey forms. For example, while an "N" for SEX might reasonably be assumed to be a mistyped "M," it is not clear whether an "R" for STUDENT refers to a "Y" or an "N." In such situations, the respondent's file must be consulted. Missing values in a computer database may also require reference back to the original survey forms. Sometimes information missing in the computer file may have been on the survey forms but overlooked by the data entry person.

	Before Cleaning		After Cleaning	
Variable	Response	Frequency	Response	Frequency
SEX	F	498	F	498
	M	493	M	496
	m	3		
	N	1		
STUDENT	N	899	N	903
	N	2	Y	89
	R	1	[Missing]	2
	Y	87		
	y	1		
	[Missing]	4		

FIGURE 25-2 **Example of Data Cleaning**

This is also the time to clean up extremely unreasonable answers. For example, suppose a participant's age in years is listed as 192. This number can reasonably be assumed to be a typo, and the original survey form should be consulted for the true age. If the survey form lists the age as 192 or if the survey was computer-assisted and there is no paper trail, then this value should be excluded from analysis because it is clearly an impossible age. However, a study of adults could reasonably include an individual with an age of 105 years. So this value would not be reasonable to delete or ignore, although it would be worth checking the original survey form for agreement with the entry in the database.

Data cleaning should also ensure that duplicate entries are removed from the database and that the records are complete, with all data from all participants entered into the database.

■ 25.4 Data Recoding

The *recoding* of variables into new categories can be done either prior to or during data analysis. Recoding prior to intense analysis is often the easiest approach when the intended new categories are known. For example, the variable AGE could be used to create a new variable for ADULT that is coded as 0 (no) for any participant younger than 18 years old and 1 (yes) for any participant age 18 or older. The variable WORK could be used to create a new variable called FULLTIME that is coded as 1 (yes) if the answer to WORK was FULLTIME and 0 (no) for any other response.

A few basic practices will help protect a cleaned data file. Never do any recoding until an original version of the cleaned data file is safely backed up elsewhere. A saved file allows a researcher to go back to the original and start anew if a file is damaged during recoding. Also, never recode into the same variable; that is, do not replace the original values with the new recoded values. Instead, always recode into a different (new) variable. Having the original variable and the new variable in the file enables the researcher to compare the original and recoded values, thus confirming that the recoding was done correctly.

■ 25.5 Maintaining Confidentiality

Chapter 23 emphasized the importance of maintaining the confidentiality of any information participants disclosed to researchers. One way to maintain confidentiality is to safely store paper records, including signed informed consent statements, in a locked and secure room. Another is to destroy individually identifying information once the records are no longer needed (such as after the data have been entered into a computer file and the files have been thoroughly cleaned) and a research ethics committee has approved the secure disposal of consent statements and other documents.

Another way to protect confidentiality is to create secure computerized data files. In general, no individually identifying information (such as a name or national identity card number) should be included in an electronic file containing other information about participants (such as responses to surveys or the results of laboratory tests). If there is a need to link records to individuals—and there is often no need to do this—then the records should be linked to identifying information by a unique study identification number. The file containing individual names should be stored in a separate and secure place, not on the same computer as the other participant data. Files containing identifiable information should be password-protected, and access to them should be limited to essential research personnel. Consult with an information technology expert or a research ethics committee if questions or concerns about securing participant information arise.

Descriptive Statistics

When employed appropriately and accurately, statistics provide essential and useful information for making sense of health research data. Descriptive statistics are used to describe the basic characteristics of study populations and other data sources.

■ 26.1 Analytic Plan by Study Approach

Statistics can be used to tell a complete and compelling story about the data collected during a research study. For most papers, and especially those written by researchers with limited experience in advanced statistics, the goal of analysis should be to use the simplest statistics possible to make the results of the study clear. Most research studies do not require the use of complex statistics like regression, and using advanced statistical tests incorrectly is, of course, never helpful.

The type of analytic plan that is commonly used with each of the major study approaches is shown in FIGURE 26-1. Each starts with a description of the study population. Studies with no comparison group, like case series and cross-sectional surveys, may need only univariate analysis. Simple statistics, like counts (frequencies), proportions, and averages, are likely to provide an adequate description of the study population. For studies that compare two or more populations—including case-control, cohort, and experimental studies—the description of the study population must be completed before moving on to bivariate analysis, such as the calculation of rate ratios, odds ratios, and other comparative statistical tests (described in Chapter 27).

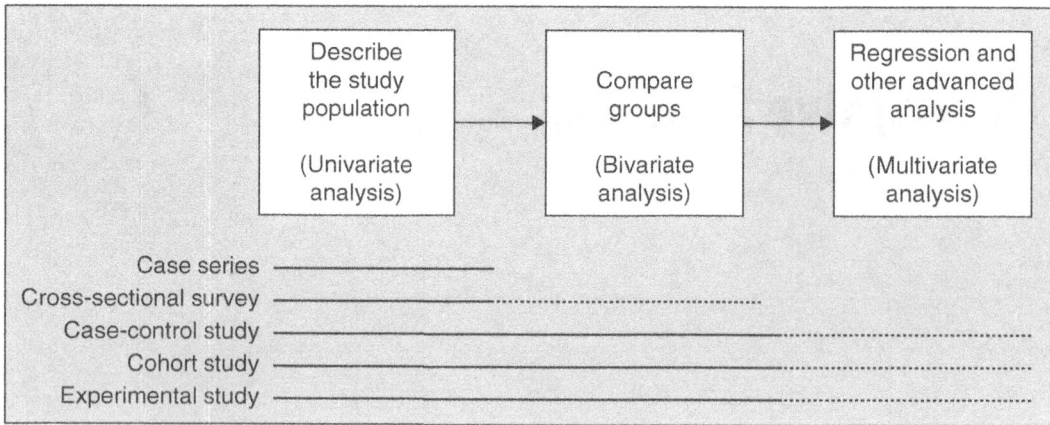

FIGURE 26-1 **Analytic Plan**

Advanced statistical analysis that examines three or more variables at one time is rarely required (and is briefly described in Chapter 28).

■ 26.2 Types of Variables

A *variable* is a characteristic that can be assigned more than one value. Examples of variables that could be examined during a population health study are age, sex, annual income, languages spoken at home, frequency of alcohol ingestion, history of chicken pox, and use of contact lenses. The value of a variable for an individual does not have to vary (change) over time, but the response among individuals within a population should be something that might differ.

In many statistical and database programs, responses from individual participants are displayed in rows with each column representing one variable. For example, one column of data may represent sex. One value for sex—an F for females or an M for males—will be listed in each row. Another column may represent age in years, and one value for age—usually a whole number—will be listed in each row.

There are several ways to classify variables (FIGURE 26-2).

- *Ratio variables* have numeric responses plotted on a scale on which a value of zero stands for "nothing." For example, if height is measured in feet, a measurement of 0 feet tall means that there was no height. As a result, the ratio of heights is meaningful. A person who is 6 feet tall is twice as tall as a person who is 3 feet tall, yielding a ratio of 2 to 1.

Variable Type	Definition	Examples
Ratio	Numbers on a scale that has a meaningful zero	Blood pressure, height, weight (If the weight increases from 10 kg to 20 kg, the weight has doubled; so the ratio of 20 kg to 10 kg is meaningful.)
Interval	Numbers on a scale that does not have a meaningful zero	Temperature (°F or °C) (The temperature does not double if it increases from 20° to 40° because 0° does not represent the absence of all heat.)
Ordinal/ranked	An ordered series that assigns a rank to responses (from first to last in the series) but for which the numbers assigned to the values are not meaningful	Highest educational degree earned, scales for never (1) to always (5), scales for strongly disagree (1) to strongly agree (5)
Nominal/categorical	Categories with no inherent rank or order	Employment category, blood type
Binomial	Nominal variables for which only two responses are possible	yes/no, male/female, case/control

FIGURE 26-2 Types of Variables

- *Interval variables* are also numeric, but they are plotted on a scale on which zero does not stand for "nothing." An outside temperature of 0°C does not mean that there is no heat; if the weather turns colder, the temperature may fall to –10°C or lower. A day with a high temperature of 40°C is not twice as hot as a day with a maximum temperature of 20°C.
- *Ordinal variables*, or *ranked variables*, order responses from first to last or from best to worst or from most favorable to least favorable. The rank order can be assigned a number. For example, the responses to a survey that asks participants to indicate their level of agreement with a statement can be coded with agree as "3," neutral as "2," and disagree as "1." Alternately, responses could be coded with agree as "1" and disagree as "3." Or neutral could be set as "0," agree as "1," and disagree as "–1." No matter what the scale is, the order of the responses is indicated by their numeric values. (Figure 18-4 provides examples of other types of ranked responses.)
- *Nominal variables*, or *categorical variables*, have categorical responses with no inherent rank or order. For example, there is no obvious way to numerically rank participants' favorite recreational sports activities or blood types. *Binomial variables* are a subtype of categorical variables with only two possible answers, usually yes and no.

Ratio and interval variables can be further classified as either continuous variables or discrete variables.

- *Continuous variables* can take on any value within a range. For example, although height is often rounded to the nearest inch when it is measured, a person's height could actually be 64½ inches or 73¾ inches or 58.1528 inches.
- *Discrete variables* typically result from counting something, so there are gaps between acceptable values. For example, a family can own 2 egg-laying chickens or 17 chickens, but cannot own 2½ chickens or 5¼ chickens.

■ 26.3 Measures of Central Tendency

Descriptive statistics are often used to describe the "average" response to a variable in a population. (For numeric variables, the average is often referred to as the *central tendency*.) There are several ways to report the average (FIGURE 26-3).

- The sample *mean* is calculated by adding up the values of all responses provided to a question and dividing that sum by the total number of individuals who answered the question.
- The *median* is the middle number when all responses are put in order from least to greatest. Half of the responses in a data set will be greater than the median, and half will be less.
- The *mode* is the most common answer given by respondents.

For ratio and interval variables, the central tendency can be described using means, medians, and modes. For ordinal variables, a median or mode can be reported. A mode can be reported for categorical variables.

Values Reported by Participants	Measure of Central Tendency	Value	Calculation
25	Mean	39.5	(25 + 30 + 30 + 40 + 50 + 62) ÷ 6
40			= 237 ÷ 6 = 39.5
30	Median	35	The two middle values from 25-30-30-40-50-62 are
50			30 and 40; 35 is halfway between 30 and 40.
30	Mode	30	Two participants provided a response of 30; no other
62			responses were listed more than once.

FIGURE 26-3 Example of a Mean, Median, and Mode

◼ 26.4 Measures of Spread

Means and medians provide information about the center of a data set, but they do not provide information about how much variability exists in the data set. For example, the participants in a study of adults with a mean age of 50 years may all be 50 years old, or they could range from 18 to 104 years old. That information is very important to have when interpreting the meaning of the results. Measures of *spread*, also called *dispersion*, are used to describe the variability and range of responses.

The *range* for a variable is the difference between the responses with the greatest and least numeric values. For example, if the youngest participant in a study is 18 years old and the oldest is 104 years old, the range is 104 − 18 = 86 years.

The median marks the value that divides the responses into two halves with equal numbers of observations. *Quartiles* mark the three values that divide a data set into four equal parts. Similarly, *tertiles* divide a data set into three equal parts, *quintiles* divide a data set into five equal parts, and *deciles* divide a data set into 10 equal parts. The *interquartile range (IQR)* is the range for the 25th to 75th percentiles, which captures the middle 50% of responses. A *boxplot* (also called a box-and-whisker plot) can be used to display this information (FIGURE 26-4). Boxplots can be especially helpful for displaying the

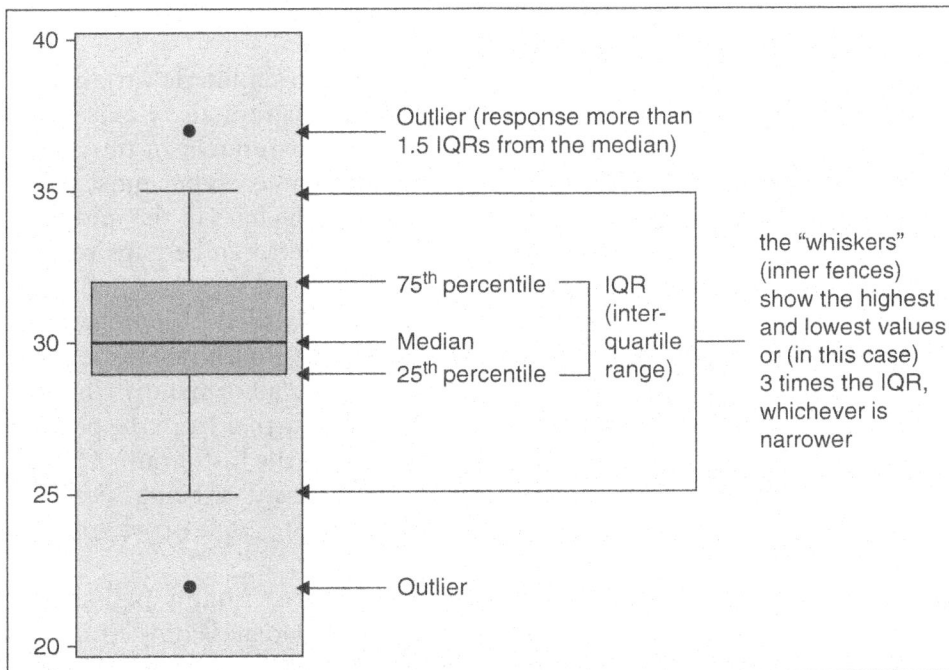

FIGURE 26-4 **Sample Boxplot**

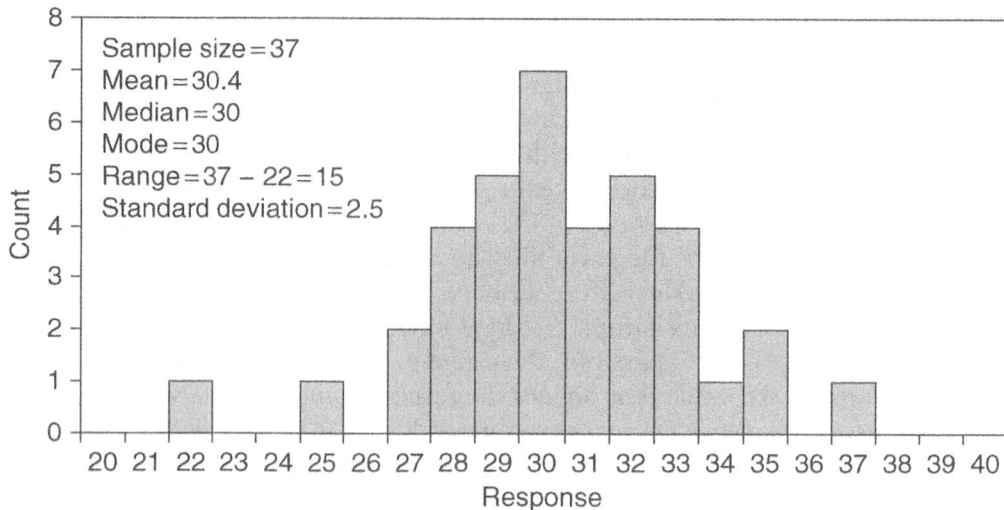

Sample size = 37
Mean = 30.4
Median = 30
Mode = 30
Range = 37 – 22 = 15
Standard deviation = 2.5

FIGURE 26-5 Sample Histogram
For the same data shown in Figure 26-4.

distribution of responses when the responses are skewed. Skewing occurs when the "whiskers" on the boxplot extend much farther on one side of the median than on the other side.

A *histogram* is an alternate way to display the responses to a numeric variable like a ratio variable or an interval variable (FIGURE 26-5). On a histogram, the *x*-axis shows the values of responses, and the *y*-axis shows the count of the number of times each response was given. For a graph to be considered a histogram, each bar must be the same width. Importantly, there should be no gaps between the bars in the middle of the distribution, where responses are clumped together. (There can be gaps to indicate values of the variable with a count of 0 responses.)

A histogram showing a *normal distribution* (*Gaussian distribution*) or *approximately normal distribution* of responses will have a bell-shaped curve with one peak in the middle (FIGURE 26-6). However, not all numeric variables have a normal distribution. The distribution may be skewed, with responses that extend farther from the peak on either the left (*left-skewed*) or the right (*right-skewed*) side of the histogram. The distribution may have a *bimodal* (two-peaked) distribution instead of being *unimodal* (one peak). Or it may be *uniform*, with about equal numbers of people providing each response.

For variables with a relatively normal distribution—a reasonably bell-shaped curve—the *standard deviation* describes the narrowness or wideness of the range of responses. When the responses are normal:

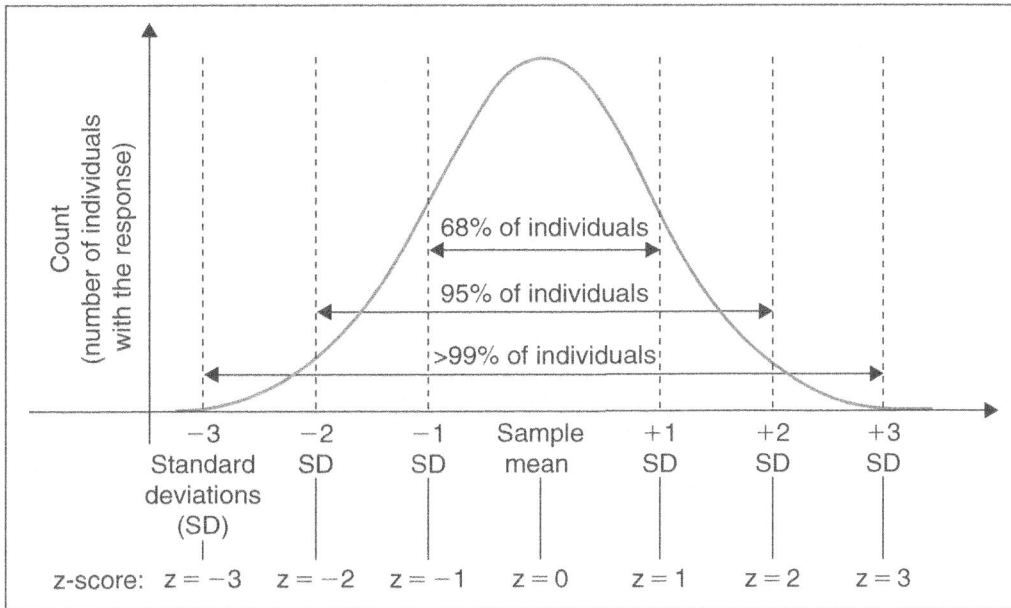

FIGURE 26-6 Example of the Distribution of Responses for a Normally Distributed Numeric Variable

- 68% of responses fall within one standard deviation above or below the mean.
- 95% of responses are within two standard deviations above or below the mean.
- More than 99% of responses are within three standard deviations above or below the mean (Figure 26-6).

A small standard deviation indicates that most responses were fairly close to the mean. A large standard deviation indicates that the range of responses was wide.

A z-*score* indicates how many standard deviations away from the sample mean an individual's response is. For example:

- An individual whose age is exactly the mean age in the population will have a z-score of 0.
- A person whose age is one standard deviation above the mean in the population will have a z-score of 1.
- A person whose age is two standard deviations below the population mean will have a z-score of –2.

A histogram or boxplot cannot be used to display the responses to categorical variables. The distribution of responses must instead be displayed in a bar chart (or, less often, a pie chart). Like a histogram, the x-axis of a *bar chart* shows the values of responses,

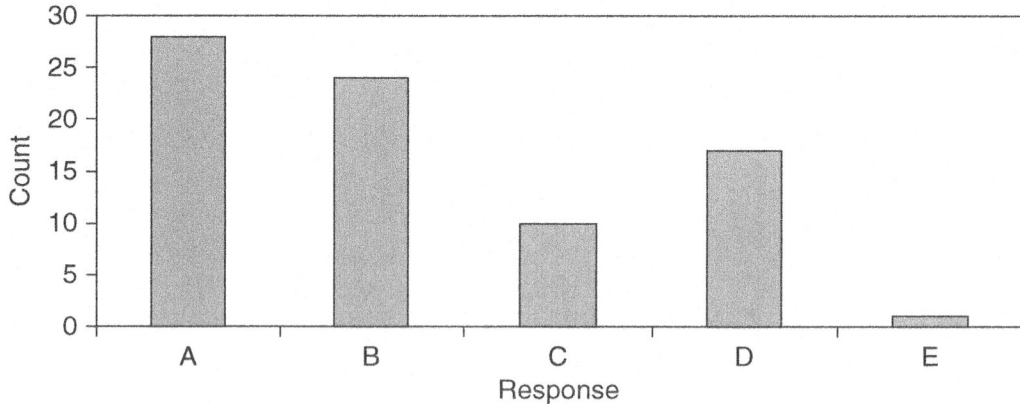

FIGURE 26-7 Sample Bar Chart

and the *y*-axis shows the count of the times each response was given. However, for a bar chart the *x*-axis can display either a number or a word. And while histograms require numbered bars to be evenly spaced along a number line, responses on bar charts may appear in any order (FIGURE 26-7). The bars in bar charts can be displayed vertically or horizontally, and there are usually spaces between the bars.

The goal of descriptive statistics is to describe accurately all the responses to a variable (FIGURE 26-8).

- For ratio and interval variables, the mean and standard deviation are typically reported.
- For ordinal variables (and for ratio and continuous variables without a normal distribution like the bell-shaped curve shown in Figure 26-6), the median and interquartile range are often reported.

Variable Type	Common Measure of Central Tendency	Common Measure of Spread	Typical Means of Display
Ratio	Mean	Standard deviation	Histogram
Interval	Mean	Standard deviation	Histogram
Ordinal/ranked	Median	Interquartile range	Boxplot
Nominal/categorical	Mode	—	Bar chart, pie chart
Binomial	Mode	—	Bar chart

FIGURE 26-8 Common Descriptive Statistics by Variable Type

- For categorical variables, the proportion of participants who provided a particular response is usually used to describe the population.

26.5 Statistical Honesty

Researchers are obligated to describe their data accurately and to correctly report the results of statistical tests. To do otherwise is a form of research misconduct. Three of the most serious forms of research misconduct are:

- Falsification—the misrepresentation of results.
- Fabrication—the creation of fake data.
- Plagiarism—the use of other people's ideas or words without proper attribution.

Statistical honesty requires more than merely avoiding outright falsification, fabrication, and plagiarism. It also requires adherence to accepted statistical practices. For example, it may be tempting to look for statistical tests that will yield the results the researcher desires, such as ones that are considered statistically significant. However, scientific integrity requires researchers to follow established statistical practices. Examples of unacceptable practices include:

- Running a dozen different types of statistical tests on a data set, hoping that one of them will happen to yield a statistically significant result to feature in a report. Instead, the researcher must select the correct test for the question being asked and the variables being examined.
- Recoding ratio variables into categorical variables by preferentially selecting the cutoff points that yield statistically significant results for tests of the new categorical variable.
- Ignoring outliers—unusual responses to a question—without a valid and standard reason. For example, a recorded birth weight of 80 pounds may be reasonably assumed to be an error in the data file, and it can be removed from analysis. But it is not reasonable to remove an 80-pound adult from the data file because an adult could weigh 80 pounds.

Statistical analysis is about discovering the true story in a data set, not about creatively manipulating data toward a preferred result.

26.6 Consultation and Collaboration

Ideally, the researcher should consult with a statistician during the study design process to ensure that:

- The sampling methods and sample size are appropriate.

- The questionnaire will yield usable data.
- The analytic strategy is a reasonable one.

Checking with an expert for the first time later in the study increases the risk of unfixable flaws in the study data. If answering the study question adequately requires the use of elaborate analytic techniques, invite an expert in that technique to serve as a collaborator and as a coauthor on the resulting paper. An invitation to collaborate should be made as early as possible in the project and in consultation with other coauthors (see Chapter 5).

Comparative Statistics

Comparative statistics compare groups of participants by sex or age, by exposure or disease status, or by other characteristics. Examples of comparative statistical tests include rate ratios, odds ratios, t-tests, and Chi-square tests. This chapter provides a brief overview of p-values, confidence intervals, and some of the most common comparative statistics used in the health sciences.

■ 27.1 Comparative Analysis by Study Approach

Some types of studies require the use of *comparative statistical tests*. These tests categorize study participants into two or more groups and compare the characteristics of

Study Approach	First Step	Key Analysis
Case-control study	Show that cases and controls are similar except for disease status	Use odds ratios (ORs) to see whether cases and controls have different exposure histories
Cohort study	Show that the exposed and unexposed are similar except for exposure status	Use rate ratios (RRs) to see whether the exposed and unexposed have different rates of incident disease
Experimental study	Show that the individuals assigned to the intervention and control groups are similar except for exposure status	Use rate ratios (RRs) and other measures to see if the intervention and control groups have different outcomes

FIGURE 27-1 Analytic Plan for Comparing Groups

the groups. For example, the analysis of a case-control study requires using comparative tests to show that the cases (people with the disease) and controls (people without the disease) in the study were similar in terms of age distribution and other demographic characteristics. Then additional comparative tests are applied to determine whether the exposure histories of cases and controls were different. Comparative tests can also be used to compare before and after characteristics of participants in longitudinal and experimental studies. FIGURE 27-1 summarizes the use of comparative statistics for several common study approaches.

■ 27.2 Hypotheses for Statistical Tests

Comparative statistical tests usually are designed to test for difference rather than for sameness. Accordingly, statistical test questions are usually phrased in terms of differences: Are the means different? Are the proportions different? Are the distributions different? Each question about statistical difference has two possible answers: The values are either different or not different.

Goal	Statistical Question	Null Hypothesis (H_0)	Alternative Hypothesis (H_a)
Test whether the average ages of cases and controls in a case-control study are similar enough to be considered equal	Are the means *different*?	The means are *not* different.	The means *are* different.
Test whether the mean age of participants drawn from a population with a mean age of 40 years is close enough to 40 years that the study population can be considered representative of the source population	Was the mean age in the study population *different* from 40 years?	The mean is *not* different from 40.	The mean *is* different from 40.
Test whether the proportion of responses to a categorical question about the frequency of flossing was similar for male and female participants in a cohort study	Are the distributions of responses *different*?	The distributions are *not* different.	The distributions *are* different.
Test whether participants, on average, had a change in their scores on a pretest administered prior to an intervention and a post-test administered after the intervention	Are the before scores of participants *different* from the after scores?	The scores are *not* different.	The scores *are* different.

FIGURE 27-2 Examples of Hypotheses for Statistical Tests

The term *null hypothesis (H₀)* describes the expected result of a statistical test if there is no difference between the two values being compared. (*Null* means nothing or zero. A *null result* means that there was no statistically significant difference.) The *alternative hypothesis (H_a)* describes the expected result if there is a difference (FIGURE 27-2). For example, for a test to compare the mean ages of two groups of study participants, the hypotheses could be as follows:

- H_0: There is *no* significant difference between the two means.
- H_a: There *is* a significant difference between the two means.

A test to compare the distribution of responses to a categorical question in two groups would have:

- H_0: There is *no* significant difference in the distribution of responses in the two populations.
- H_a: There *is* a significant difference in the distribution of responses in the two populations.

◼ 27.3 Rejecting the Null Hypothesis

Because statistical tests do not ask questions about sameness, the answers provided by statistical tests do not allow a researcher to say conclusively whether two values are the same. Instead, a researcher must make a conclusion about whether the results of a statistical test indicate that values are different or not different. The language used to describe this decision is that the researcher will either "reject the null hypothesis" or "fail to reject the null hypothesis."

- *Rejecting the null hypothesis* means concluding that the values are different by rejecting the claim that the values are not different.
- *Failing to reject the null hypothesis* means concluding that there is no evidence that the values are different. Functionally, this is like saying that the values are close enough to be considered similar, but failing to reject the null hypothesis should never be taken as evidence that the values are the same.

The decision to reject or fail to reject the null hypothesis is based on the likelihood that the result of a test was due to chance. One way to understand the concept of chance is to consider the variability in sample populations. When a sample population is drawn from a source population, the mean age in the sample population is usually not exactly the mean age of the source population. (See Figure 17-1 for an illustration of the variety of sample means that can occur in different samples drawn from one source population.) The range of expected values for the mean age of sample populations drawn from a source population can be estimated using statistics (FIGURE 27-3). Some sample populations will have mean ages that are very close to the mean in the

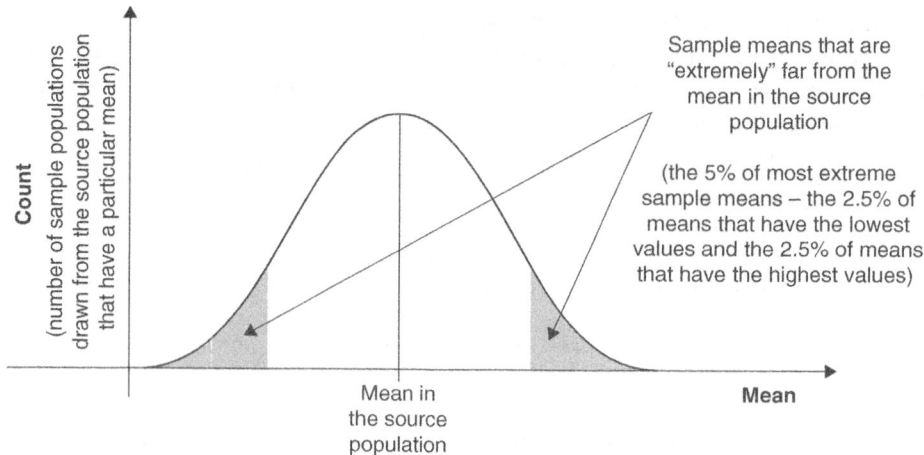

FIGURE 27-3 **Example of the Distribution of Mean Ages for Sample Populations Drawn from a Larger Source Population**

source population; other sample populations will have mean ages that are quite far from the mean in the source population. No set cutoff defines what will be considered extremely far from the mean age in the source population, but the standard is to say that the 5% of sample means farthest from the true mean are extreme. Thus, by chance, 5% of the samples drawn from a source population will be expected to have an extreme mean.

Similarly, if two sample populations are drawn from the same source population, their mean ages will not be identical even though they are drawn from the same pool of individuals. Comparative statistical tests accommodate this expected difference when testing whether two groups in a study population are different. For example, a test that compares the mean ages of cases and controls in a case-control study adjusts for the fact that there will be some difference between the mean ages of cases and controls, even if the cases and controls are sampled from source populations with identical mean ages. The test will also examine whether the mean ages are so far apart that, if the cases and controls were drawn from source populations with the same mean age, the difference between the mean ages of the cases and the controls would fall in the 5% of most extreme differences expected by chance.

When the difference in mean ages is great, the statistical test will show that it is highly unlikely that the group means are not significantly different. The researcher will therefore reject the null hypothesis and conclude that the mean ages of the cases and the controls are different. The difference between the mean ages of cases and controls will be taken as evidence that the mean age of individuals in the source population for cases and the mean age of individuals in the source population for controls are different. This conclusion assumes that the difference between the source populations is reflected in the sample of cases and controls that happened to be drawn from their respective source populations.

If the statistical test shows that the mean ages of cases and controls are fairly close, the researcher will fail to reject the null hypothesis and will conclude that the means are not different.

■ 27.4 Interpreting *p*-Values

A p-*value*, or *probability value*, for a statistical test is used to decide whether the results observed are likely to reflect real differences between groups. The interpretation is similar for all statistical tests: the *p*-value for the study determines whether the null hypothesis (H_0) will be rejected. The standard is to use a *significance level* of $\alpha = 0.05$, or 5%. Any statistical test with a result that is in the 5% of most extreme responses expected by chance will result in the rejection of the null hypothesis (FIGURE 27-4). Alternatively, some studies use $\alpha = 0.01$, which makes it harder for a test to find a statistically significant result that would cause the rejection of the null hypothesis. Others use $\alpha = 0.10$, which makes it more likely that a test will yield a statistically significant result.

Some *p*-values are reported as being one-sided or two-sided, based on the alternative hypothesis for the statistical test. While most statistical tests use an alternative hypothesis that simply expresses difference (such as "the means are different"), some tests allow for an alternative hypothesis that states the direction of the difference (like "males have a higher mean age than females") (FIGURE 27-5). If a direction is specified in the alternative hypothesis, then all of the extreme values (all of the shaded area shown in Figure 27-3) will be on one side of the distribution (either all on the left of the distribution or all on the right). When this direction is specified, a one-sided *p*-value can be

H_0	Conclusion When . . .	
	$p < 0.05^* =$ reject H_0	$p \geq 0.05^* =$ fail to reject H_0
The means are not different.	The means are different.	The means are not different.
The proportions are not different.	The proportions are different.	The proportions are not different.
The distributions are not different.	The distributions are different.	The distributions are not different.

*Assuming $\alpha = 0.05$.

FIGURE 27-4 Interpreting *p*-Values

Null Hypothesis (H$_0$)	Two-Sided Alternative Hypothesis (H$_a$)	Example of a One-Sided Alternative Hypothesis (H$_a$)
The means are not different.	The means are different.	The mean of cases is higher than the mean of controls.
The proportions are not different.	The proportions are different.	The proportion of the intervention group is lower than the proportion of the control group.
The scores are not different.	The scores are different.	The after scores were, on average, higher than the before scores.

FIGURE 27-5 Examples of One-Sided and Two-Sided Alternative Hypotheses

used. In all other situations a two-sided p-value should be used to make the decision about rejecting or failing to reject the null hypothesis.

■ 27.5 Interpreting Confidence Intervals

Confidence intervals (CIs) provide information about the expected value of a measure in a source population based on the value of that measure in a study population (FIGURE 27-6). For example, if the mean age in a study population of 1000 people sampled from a large city is 30 years, a researcher should not assume that the mean age in the whole city is exactly 30 years. The 95% confidence interval states how close to 30 years the mean age in the source population (the whole city) is expected to be. If the 95% confidence interval for the mean age in the study population extends from 28 to 32, a researcher can be 95% confident that the mean age in the city is between 28 and 32 years.

The width of the interval is related to the sample size of the study. A larger sample size will yield a narrower confidence interval. If every member of the source population is included in the study population, then a confidence interval is not needed because the exact value for the source population will be known.

A 95% confidence interval is usually reported, and that corresponds to a significance level of $\alpha = 0.05$ for a statistical test. This means that 5% of the time a 95% confidence interval is expected to miss capturing the true value of a measure in the source population. Using a 99% confidence interval ($\alpha = 0.01$) would make the confidence interval wider and make it more likely that the value in the source population would be captured within the confidence interval. But it would also make it more difficult to classify a result as statistically significant because fewer results would be classified as extreme. Alternatively, a 90% confidence interval ($\alpha = 0.10$) could be used. A 90% confidence interval would be narrower and make it easier for a result to be deemed statistically significant because more results would be classified as extreme. However, a 90% confidence interval would be less likely than a 95% confidence interval to

Statistic	Result with 95% CI	Interpretation
Mean age of all participants (years)	30 (28, 32)	Based on the mean age in the study population (30 years), we are 95% confident that the mean age in the source population is between 28 and 32 years.
Proportion of all participants with a disease (%)	9.0 (7.3, 10.9)	Based on the proportion of individuals in the study population who had the disease (9.0%), we are 95% confident that the prevalence of disease in the source population is between 7.3% and 10.9%.
Odds ratio (OR)	1.7 (0.6, 5.3)	Based on the OR in the study population (OR = 1.7), we are 95% confident that the OR in the source population is somewhere between 0.6 and 5.3. Because this overlaps with OR = 1, we conclude that there is no association between the exposure and disease status.
Relative risk (RR)	1.6 (1.1, 2.4)	Based on the RR in the study population (RR = 1.6), we are 95% confident that the RR in the source population is between 1.1 and 2.4. Because this range does not overlap with RR = 1, we conclude that the exposure is associated with an increased risk of disease.

FIGURE 27-6 Interpreting Confidence Intervals (CIs)

capture the true value in the source population. For example, a 90% confidence interval for an odds ratio (OR) is less likely to overlap with OR = 1 than a 99% confidence interval. So, although the 90% confidence interval is less likely to capture the true odds ratio, it is also more likely that the OR will be deemed to show a statistically significant association between the exposure and the outcome (FIGURE 27-7).

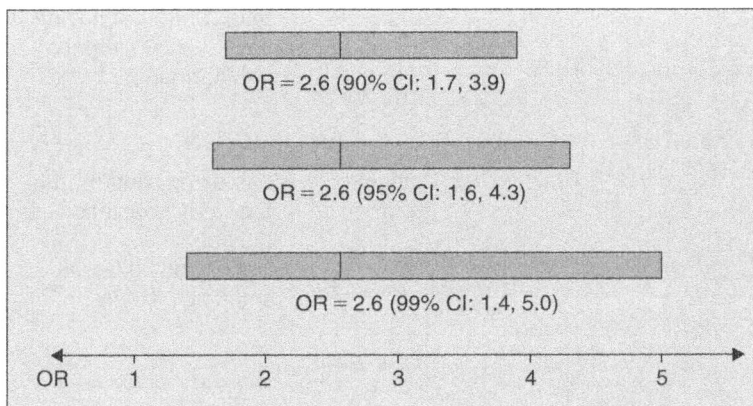

OR = 2.6 (90% CI: 1.7, 3.9)

OR = 2.6 (95% CI: 1.6, 4.3)

OR = 2.6 (99% CI: 1.4, 5.0)

OR   1   2   3   4   5

FIGURE 27-7 90%, 95%, and 99% Confidence Intervals (CIs) for the Same Odds Ratio (OR)

■ 27.6 Measures of Association

Some of the most common types of comparative analysis are the measures of association explained in the chapters on the various study approaches, such as the correlation used for ecological studies (Chapter 8), the odds ratio (OR) used for case-control studies (Chapter 11), and the rate ratio (RR) used for cohort studies (Chapter 12).

The OR and RR compare responses to two variables that have each been divided into two levels using what is sometimes called *2x2 analysis*. Prior to using a computer to calculate an OR or RR, variables that are not already divided into two categories must be recoded into binomial variables (often coded numerically as yes = 1 and no = 0). In some situations, the cutoff points for the categories are obvious, such as those that divide an ordinal variable into categories for disagreement (strongly disagree or disagree) and agreement (agree or strongly agree). Sometimes the population can be divided into groups of relatively equal sizes using the median, quartiles, or other sample-based cutoff points. Alternatively, biologically or socially meaningful cutoff points can be defined, such as using the 18th birthday to divide a study population into children and adults. The choice of cutoff point will influence whether the

Exposure		Percentage of Cases (AMI) ($n = 150$)	Percentage of Controls (no AMI) ($n = 250$)	OR (95% CI)	Interpretation
Sex	Female	39.3%	42.4%	Reference group	Cases and controls in the study did *not* have significantly different proportions of males.
	Male	60.7%	57.6%	1.14 (0.75, 1.72)	
Waist circumference >35 inches	no	37.3%	51.2%	Reference group	Cases had greater odds than controls of having a waist circumference greater than 35 inches.
	yes	62.7%	48.8%	1.76 (1.16, 2.67)*	
Tobacco use	Never smoked	68.0%	73.6%	Reference group	Cases and controls in the study population did *not* have significantly different smoking histories.
	Former smoker	11.3%	10.8%	1.14 (0.58, 2.18)	
	Current smoker	20.7%	15.6%	1.43 (0.84, 2.44)	

*Statistically significant at $\alpha = 0.05$ level.

FIGURE 27-8 Example of Odds Ratios for a Case-Control Study of Acute Myocardial Infarction

exposure and outcome have a statistically significant association. Accordingly, the decision about how to define categories should be justifiable.

The results of 2×2 analysis are often presented using tables like the one shown in FIGURE 27-8. The reference group for an odds ratio or rate ratio should be well defined. In the example, males are compared to females, those with a waist circumference greater than 35 inches to those with smaller girths, former smokers to never smokers, and current smokers to never smokers. (Two separate odds ratios were calculated for tobacco use because the variable for tobacco use had three possible responses instead of just two.)

The 95% confidence interval provides information about the statistical significance of the tests. For example, the 95% confidence interval for the odds ratio comparing the sex distribution of cases and controls contains OR = 1. This means that it is not clear from the test whether cases are more likely or less likely than controls to be male. The conclusion is therefore that there is no statistically significant difference in the proportion of cases and controls by sex.

■ 27.7 Selecting an Appropriate Test

For statistical comparisons more complex than 2×2 analysis, analysts must select a test that is appropriate to the goal of the analysis and the types of variables being analyzed. The steps for identifying and using a statistical test are summarized in FIGURE 27-9.

First, the variables to be compared should be selected and the goal of the test clearly stated. The goal could be:

- To compare the mean ages of males and females (variables: age, sex).
- To see whether the proportion of cases and controls with various blood types is similar (variables: blood type, disease status).
- To determine whether individuals starting an exercise program had, on average, lower heart rates one month after starting the program than they did when they enrolled (variables: initial heart rate, heart rate after one month).

Then select a test that is appropriate for the types of variables being examined. Some tests require the variables being examined to have particular distributions or other characteristics. The researcher must confirm that the variables meet these *assumptions* of the test prior to running it and interpreting the output.

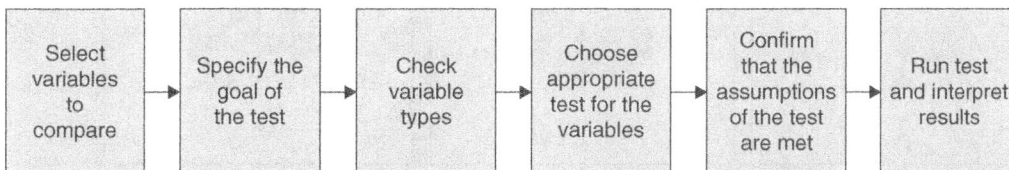

FIGURE 27-9 **Plan for Hypothesis Testing**

Statistical tests are often classified as being either parametric or nonparametric. The basic difference between these two types of tests is that parametric tests make more assumptions about the variables being examined than nonparametric tests.

- *Parametric tests* assume that the variables being examined have particular distributions, often requiring the variables to have normal or approximately normal distributions. These tests may also require that the variance for the variable of interest—the spread of observations around the mean—be equal or at least similar in the population groups being compared.
- *Nonparametric tests* do not make assumptions about the distributions of responses.

Parametric tests are typically used for ratio and interval variables with relatively normal (bell-shaped) distributions of responses. Most parametric tests are more statistically powerful than nonparametric tests. So the preference is to use a parametric test whenever the variable being examined fits reasonably well with the assumptions the test makes about sample size, distribution, and the equality of variances.

Nonparametric tests are often used for ranked variables, such as the responses to surveys that ask participants to indicate preferences using scales from 1 (strongly disagree) to 5 (strongly agree). They are also used when the distribution of a ratio or interval variable is non-normal. Additionally, nonparametric tests are used for categorical variables, including variables with just two groups (such as cases and controls, males and females, children and adults).

■ 27.8 Comparing a Population to a Set Value

The goal of some statistical tests is to compare the value of a statistic in a study population to some set value. For example, suppose that participants in an experimental study are students at a university at which the mean age of undergraduate students is 21 years. The researcher wants to confirm that the mean age of the study participants is reasonably close to 21 years. If the distribution of ages in the study population looks like the distribution in Box A of FIGURE 27-10, then 21 years is captured within two

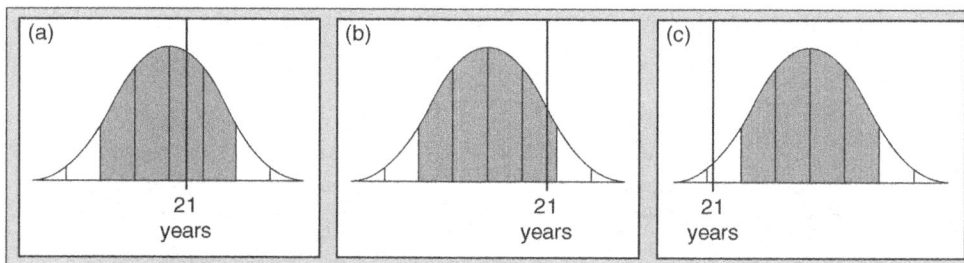

FIGURE 27-10 Comparing the Sample Mean to Some Other Value (One-Sample *t*-Test)

standard deviations of the study's mean age. The conclusion would be that the sample mean is not so far from 21 that the means would be considered different. In other words, the sample shown in Box A fails to reject the null hypothesis that the means are not different. The conclusion is that the means in the study population and the university student population as a whole are not significantly different. Box B also captures 21 years within the 95% confidence interval, even though the mean age of study participants is farther from 21 than it was in Box A. In Box C, however, the study participants were several years older than the average student at the university, and 21 years does not fall within the 95% confidence interval. This indicates that the study population may not be adequately representative of the university's undergraduate student population. In this situation, the null hypothesis is rejected, and the conclusion is that the means are different.

■ 27.9 Comparing Independent Populations

Sometimes study participants are grouped into *independent populations*, which are populations in which each individual can be a member of only one of the population groups being compared. For example, if the populations being compared are divided by age, the population of adults ages 18 to 49 will not overlap with the population of adults ages 50 to 99. Each individual participant in the study population can be assigned to, at most, one of these groups. So the populations are considered independent.

	Type of Variable Being Examined			
	Ratio/Interval (Parametric Tests)	Ordinal/Rank (Nonparametric Tests)	Binomial	Nominal Categories
Statistic being evaluated	Mean	Median	Proportion	Proportions
Test for whether the statistic in one population is different from a hypothetical value	One-sample t-test	One-sample median test	Binomial test	Chi-square (χ^2) goodness-of-fit test
Test for whether the statistic differs in two populations	Independent-samples (two-sample) t-test	Mann-Whitney U test (Wilcoxon rank sum test, Wilcoxon-Mann-Whitney test)	Fisher's exact test	Chi-square (χ^2) test
Test for whether the statistic differs in two or more populations	One-way ANOVA (F-test)	Kruskal-Wallis test	Chi-square (χ^2) test	Chi-square (χ^2) test

FIGURE 27-11 Tests for Comparing Two or More Groups

Variable	Report	Males ($n = 200$)	Females ($n = 200$)	Variable Type	Test of Comparison	p-value for Test	Interpretation
Age	Mean (SD)	43.7 (7.8)	41.1 (8.1)	Ratio (normal)	Independent-samples t-test	0.001	The means are different.
Current smokers	%	12.0%	9.5%	Binomial (yes / no)	Fisher's exact test	0.519	The proportions are *not* different.
Home district: North Central South	n (%) 90 (45.0%) 50 (25.0%) 60 (30.0%)	 87 (43.5%) 48 (24.0%) 65 (32.5%)	Nominal	Chi-square (χ^2) test	0.864	The proportions are *not* different.

FIGURE 27-12 Examples of Tests for Comparing Males and Females in a Study Population

A variety of statistical tests can be used to compare independent populations. The appropriate test to use depends on the type of variable being examined (FIGURE 27-11). For example, a two-sample (independent-samples) t-test could be used to compare the mean ages of cases and controls participating in a case-control study. A Fisher's exact test could be used to examine whether the proportions of males in the exposed and unexposed groups of a cohort study are similar. A Chi-square test could be used to determine whether the distributions of participants by race or ethnicity are similar for the intervention and control groups of an experimental study.

When running statistical tests, it is often beneficial to create a table of basic information about the variables of interest for each of the comparison groups as well as the result of the statistical tests used to compare those populations. FIGURE 27-12 shows sample output for tests of whether responses differed for the male and female participants of a cohort study. In this example, the males have a significantly greater average age than the females because the p-value for the independent-samples t-test is less than 0.05. However, the proportion of males and females who smoke is not significantly different because the p-value for Fisher's exact test was greater than 0.05.

Characteristic		Males ($n = 200$)	Females ($n = 200$)	p-value
Age	Mean (SD)	43.7 (7.8)	41.1 (8.1)	0.001*
Current smokers	%	12.0%	9.5%	0.519
Home district: North Central South	n (%)	 90 (45.0%) 50 (25.0%) 60 (30.0%)	 87 (43.5%) 48 (24.0%) 65 (32.5%)	0.864

*Statistically significant at $\alpha = 0.05$ level.
FIGURE 27-13 Simplified Version of Figure 27-12

The table shown in Figure 27-12 includes more information than is usually included in published manuscripts. However, it allows the researcher to double-check that the correct tests were used and that the correct interpretations were made. It also facilitates the writing of the statistical methods portion of the methods section of a research report. A more succinct comparison table is usually prepared for the final report. A sample results table is shown in FIGURE 27-13.

■ 27.10 Comparing Paired Data

A different set of tests is used when the goal is to compare before-and-after results in the same individuals (FIGURE 27-14). If the goal is to see whether, on average, a participant in a cohort study gained weight between the baseline exam and the 1-year follow-up exam, a matched-pairs *t*-test can be used. If the goal is to see whether a safe driving course improves the pass rates for a driving licensure exam, McNemar's test can be used to examine how many participants switched from failing a pretest to passing a post-test, how many switched from passing a pretest to failing a post-test, and how many had no change in status. McNemar's test can also determine whether the differences indicate that the course had a significant impact on exam pass rates.

FIGURE 27-15 shows sample output for paired tests. In this example, participants in a 3-month exercise program lost weight during the study period because the *p*-value for the matched-pairs *t*-test was less than 0.05, but the participants did not increase their ability to run 1 mile in less than 10 minutes. The *p*-value for McNemar's test was greater than 0.05, which indicates that there was no difference in this variable during the study period.

	Type of Variable Being Examined			
	Ratio/Interval (Parametric Tests)	Ordinal/Rank (Nonparametric Tests)	Binomial	Nominal Categories
Test for whether the value of the variable is different in one population measured twice (such as before-and-after in the same population) or in two paired groups	Matched-pairs (paired) *t*-test	Wilcoxon (matched-pairs) signed-rank test or sign test for matched pairs	McNemar's test	McNemar's test
Test for whether the value of the variable is different in two or more matched groups	One-way repeated-measures ANOVA	Friedman test	Cochran's Q test	Cochran's Q test

FIGURE 27-14 **Tests for Comparing Matched Populations**

Variable	Report	Pretest	Post-Test	Difference	Variable Type	Test of Comparison	p-Value for Test	Interpretation
Sample size	n	40	40	0	Count	–	–	–
Weight (pounds)	Mean (SD)	177.9 (18.8)	171.5 (18.6)	–6.5 (5.7)	Ratio (normal)	Matched-pairs t-test	<0.001	The pre- and post-test weights for individuals were, on average, significantly different.
Able to run 1 mile in less than 10 minutes	n (%)	12 (30%)	16 (40%)	6 no-to-yes, 2 yes-to-no, 32 no change	Binomial	McNemar's test	0.289	The pre- and post-test ability for an individual participant to run 1 mile in less than 10 minutes was, on average, *not* different.

FIGURE 27-15 Examples of Tests for Comparing Pretest and Post-Test Results for Participants in a 3-Month Exercise Program

A Brief Guide to Advanced Health Statistics

Only a very limited number of studies require regression analysis or any of the other advanced statistics that are described in this chapter. User-friendly statistical software programs have made it possible for nearly everyone to run advanced statistical analyses, but these programs still require the user to select appropriate tests and decipher what the output means. Researchers should not use these tests without first knowing when to use them, what conditions have to be met to make their use appropriate, how to run them, and how to interpret them. This chapter provides a quick reference to some of the most commonly used advanced statistical techniques.

■ 28.1 Confounding and Effect Modification

One of the main reasons researchers use multivariate statistical models—that is, analyses of three or more variables at one time—is to examine the interactions that may occur among variables. This can be especially helpful when a *third variable* (also called an extraneous variable or *lurking variable*) may be concealing or distorting the true relationship between two other variables. Several different types of *third variable effects* might occur, including confounding and effect modification.

A *confounder* may make the association between an exposure variable and an outcome variable appear more or less significant than it truly is. For example, the crude (unadjusted) odds ratio for the relationship between physical inactivity and a first heart attack may show that inactive adults are four times more likely than active adults to have a heart attack. Yet age may confound this association because older adults are more likely than younger adults to be inactive and also more likely to have a heart attack. Age-specific analysis may show that inactive young adults are twice as likely as active young adults to have a heart attack. It might also show that inactive older adults are twice as likely as active older adults to have a heart attack. These results for analysis stratified by age would indicate that age was confounding the association between exercise and heart attacks. When a third variable is shown to be a confounder, an adjusted measure of association, such as an age-adjusted odds ratio, should be reported for the association between the exposure and the outcome. In the example, instead of reporting a crude odds ratio of OR = 4, it would be more accurate to report an age-adjusted odds ratio of OR = 2.

An *effect modifier* (sometimes called an "interaction term") is a third variable that often represents biologically distinct groups of individuals who might experience different biological responses to various exposures. For example, menopausal status may be an effect modifier for some studies related to women's reproductive health issues. A particular exposure may be associated with a decreased risk of breast cancer in premenopausal women but be associated with an increased risk of breast cancer in postmenopausal women. If a third variable is shown to be an effect modifier, it is usually best to report separate stratum-specific measures of association for each level of the effect modifier (such as separate results for premenopausal and postmenopausal women). Pooling the results for the biologically different groups may hide meaningful differences, so an adjusted or crude measure of association should not be reported when effect modification is occurring.

FIGURE 28-1 summarizes the steps required to identify confounders and effect modifiers. To be a confounder or effect modifier, the third variable must be independently associated with both an exposure (or predictor) variable and an outcome variable.

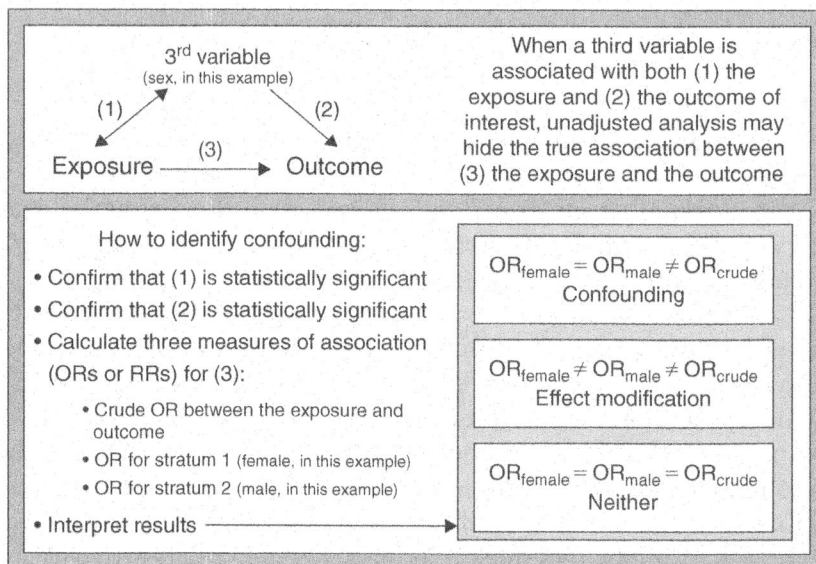

FIGURE 28-1 Confounding and Effect Modification

These two relationships should be confirmed. Then a crude odds ratio (or other measure of association) for the relationship between the exposure and the outcome should be calculated, along with a separate measure of association for each level of the third variable, such as separate odds ratios for males and females. The crude and stratum-specific measures are compared using a Breslow-Day test for homogeneity or interaction, a −2 log likelihood test, or another appropriate statistical test. After running a suitable test, the interpretation is as follows:

- If the crude and stratum-specific odds ratios are all similar, then neither confounding nor effect modification is occurring. Report a crude measure.
- If the stratum-specific measures of association are equivalent to one another but different from the crude measure of association, the third variable is a confounder. Report an adjusted measure.
- If the stratum-specific measures of association are different from one another and different from the crude measure of association, the third variable is an effect modifier. Report stratum-specific measures.

■ 28.2 Regression

Regression is often the easiest way to adjust for one or more confounding variables or interaction terms during analysis. *Regression models* seek to understand the relationship between one or more *predictor (independent) variables* and one *outcome (dependent) variable*. The models allow the effect of one predictor variable on the outcome to be examined while controlling for other predictor variables (that is, while keeping their values constant). The two most common types of regression are linear regression and logistic regression, which are discussed in the following sections. The steps for model fitting are similar for both types of models and are summarized in FIGURE 28-2.

Some statistical software programs require the analyst to:

- Select a variety of specifications for the model, such as the particular estimation technique (often an ordinary least squares, generalized least squares, or maximum likelihood estimation model).
- Choose the method the computer will use to select variables for inclusion in the model. For example, an "enter" method will include all predictor variables in the model. A "forward stepwise" method adds the best predictor variables to the model one at a time until adding an additional variable does not significantly improve the fit of the model. A "backward stepwise" method deletes variables from the model until deleting a variable significantly reduces the fit of the model.
- Check the fit of the model by examining its residual terms, which measure how well real data match the values predicted by the model, and the results of statistical tests of the goodness-of-fit for the model.

Step	
1	Select one outcome (dependent) variable.
2	Identify the appropriate type of regression (such as a linear or logistic model) for the outcome variable.
3	Select one or more predictor (independent) variables.
4	Check to make sure that any assumptions required for the model (such as the variable types or distributions of outcome and predictor variables) are met.
5	Choose a selection method for helping the computer to decide which set of predictor variables will produce the "best-fit" model (the model that the computer determines is the best at explaining the relationship between the predictor variables and the outcome variable).
6	Examine the model for potential problems. For example, examine residuals for possible autocorrelation, check for possible interaction between predictor variables (such as the multicollinearity that might occur when two predictor variables are highly correlated), and look for other potential problems that might need to be addressed.
7	Interpret the results of the regression model, and consider whether they are logical (for example, that all necessary covariates are included and all illogical ones are excluded).

FIGURE 28-2 **Steps in Fitting a Regression Model**

A statistics reference or a statistician should be consulted for detailed information about these and other advanced analytic techniques.

28.3 Linear Regression

A linear regression model is used when the outcome variable is a ratio or interval variable.

Simple linear regression models examine whether there is a linear relationship between one predictor variable and the outcome variable. FIGURE 28-3 provides an example of how to interpret the results of a simple linear regression. The relationship between the predictor and outcome variables can be visually displayed using a scatterplot, and the regression model finds the best-fit line for those points. The slope of the line is the coefficient for the predictor variable (often designated as β in the output of statistical software programs). The y-intercept for the line is the coefficient for the constant in the regression model.

These values can be used to write an equation for the best-fit line, and that equation can be used to predict the expected value of the outcome variable for various values of the predictor variable. The r^2 for the model, which is the square of the correlation

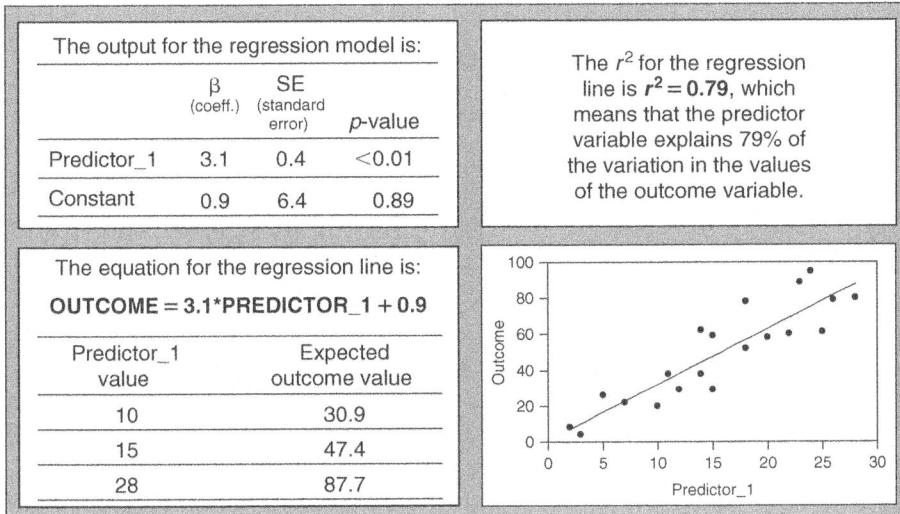

The output for the regression model is:

	β (coeff.)	SE (standard error)	p-value
Predictor_1	3.1	0.4	<0.01
Constant	0.9	6.4	0.89

The r^2 for the regression line is $r^2 = 0.79$, which means that the predictor variable explains 79% of the variation in the values of the outcome variable.

The equation for the regression line is:

OUTCOME = 3.1*PREDICTOR_1 + 0.9

Predictor_1 value	Expected outcome value
10	30.9
15	47.4
28	87.7

FIGURE 28-3 Example of a Simple Linear Regression Model

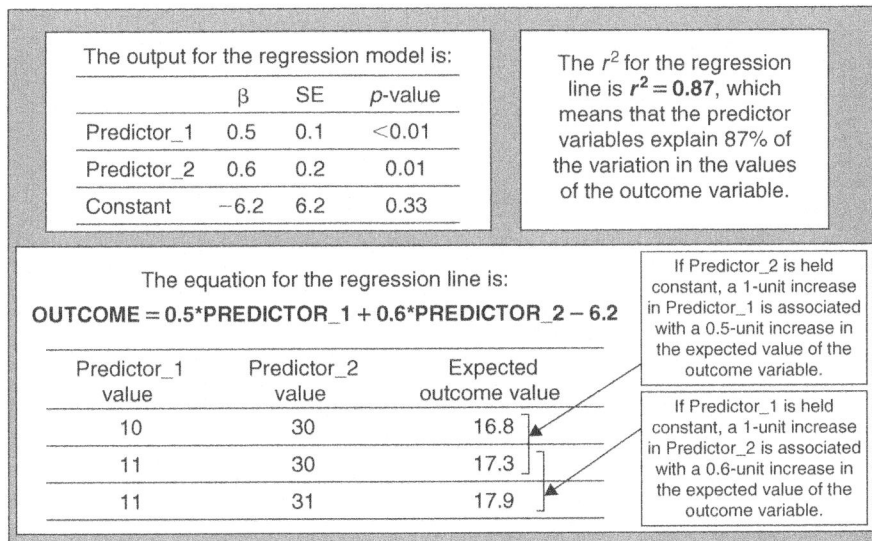

The output for the regression model is:

	β	SE	p-value
Predictor_1	0.5	0.1	<0.01
Predictor_2	0.6	0.2	0.01
Constant	−6.2	6.2	0.33

The r^2 for the regression line is $r^2 = 0.87$, which means that the predictor variables explain 87% of the variation in the values of the outcome variable.

The equation for the regression line is:

OUTCOME = 0.5*PREDICTOR_1 + 0.6*PREDICTOR_2 − 6.2

Predictor_1 value	Predictor_2 value	Expected outcome value
10	30	16.8
11	30	17.3
11	31	17.9

If Predictor_2 is held constant, a 1-unit increase in Predictor_1 is associated with a 0.5-unit increase in the expected value of the outcome variable.

If Predictor_1 is held constant, a 1-unit increase in Predictor_2 is associated with a 0.6-unit increase in the expected value of the outcome variable.

FIGURE 28-4 Example of a Multiple Linear Regression Model with Two Continuous Variables

coefficient, provides information about how well the regression model predicts the variation in the values of the outcome variable. The value of r^2 ranges from 0 to 1, with larger values indicating a better model fit.

Multiple linear regression models examine the effects of several predictor variables on the value of the outcome variable. FIGURE 28-4 provides an example of how to interpret the output for a multiple linear regression with two continuous predictor variables. The coefficients (β) for the predictor variables and the constant can be used to write an equation for a best-fit line. That equation can be used to examine the effect of each predictor variable on the outcome variable while controlling the other predictors by holding their values constant.

Multiple linear regression models can have both continuous and categorical predictor variables, as long as the responses to categorical variables are expressed by numbers. FIGURE 28-5 shows how to interpret models with multiple types of predictor variables that do not interact. In the example, a 1-unit increase in the value of the "Predictor_2" variable is associated with a 2-unit increase in the value of the outcome (since the coefficient for "Predictor_2" is $\beta = 2.0$). This relationship between "Predictor_2" and the outcome is the same for both males and females, even though males have an 18.7- unit higher value for the outcome than females (since the coefficient for sex is $\beta = 18.7$).

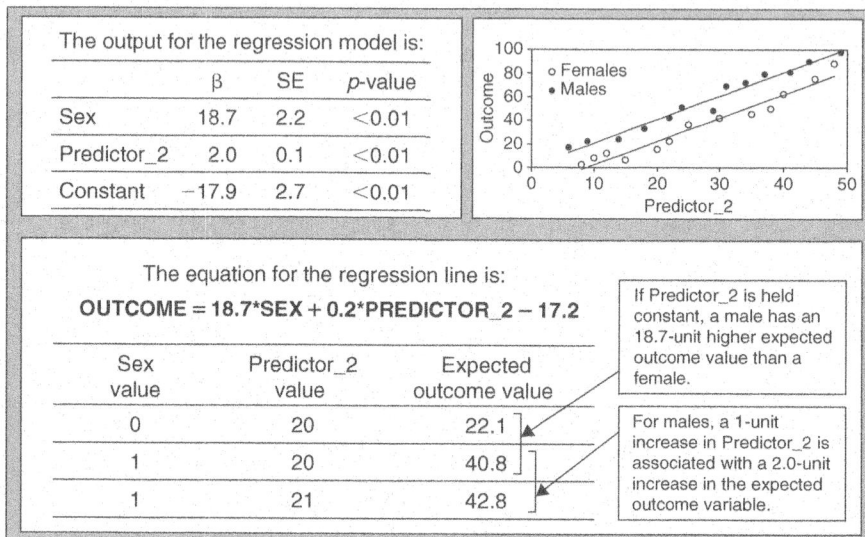

FIGURE 28-5 Example of a Multiple Linear Regression Model with One Continuous and One Categorical Variable with No Interaction (As Indicated by the Parallel Lines for Females and Males on the Graph)

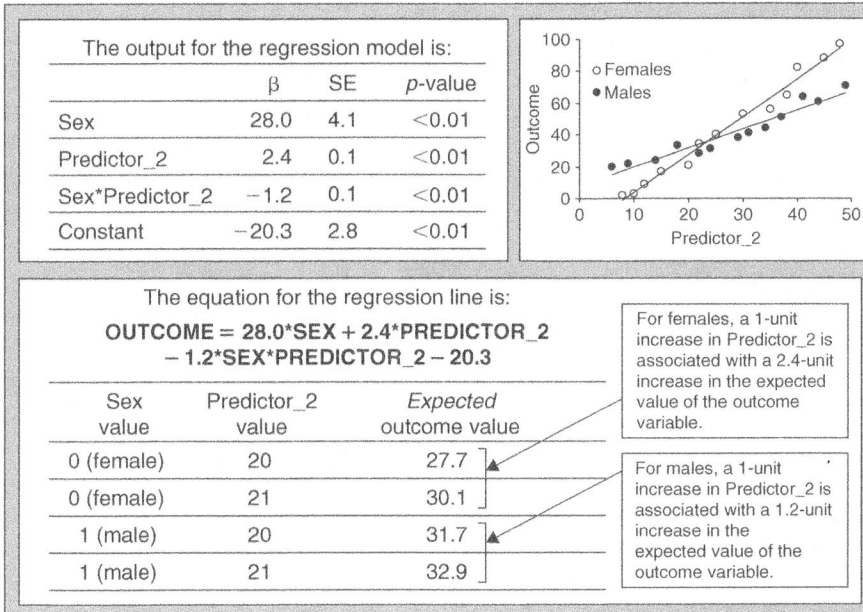

The output for the regression model is:

	β	SE	p-value
Sex	28.0	4.1	<0.01
Predictor_2	2.4	0.1	<0.01
Sex*Predictor_2	−1.2	0.1	<0.01
Constant	−20.3	2.8	<0.01

The equation for the regression line is:

OUTCOME = 28.0*SEX + 2.4*PREDICTOR_2 − 1.2*SEX*PREDICTOR_2 − 20.3

Sex value	Predictor_2 value	*Expected outcome value*
0 (female)	20	27.7
0 (female)	21	30.1
1 (male)	20	31.7
1 (male)	21	32.9

For females, a 1-unit increase in Predictor_2 is associated with a 2.4-unit increase in the expected value of the outcome variable.

For males, a 1-unit increase in Predictor_2 is associated with a 1.2-unit increase in the expected value of the outcome variable.

FIGURE 28-6 Example of a Multiple Linear Regression Model with One Continuous and One Categorical Variable with Interaction (As Indicated by the Non-parallel Lines for Males and Females on the Graph)

The predictor variables in multiple linear regression models may interact. For example, interaction may be occurring when the best-fit regression lines for males and females have considerably different slopes. FIGURE 28-6 shows how to interpret models when interaction is occurring between some of the predictor variables. In the example, a 1-unit increase in the value of the Predictor_2 variable is associated with a 2.4-unit increase in the value of the outcome for females but only a 1.2-unit increase for males. The equation for the regression model expresses this interaction through the use of a special interaction term.

■ 28.4 Logistic Regression

Logistic regression models (sometimes called logit regression models) are used when the outcome variable is a dichotomous variable. Logistic regression is commonly used in case-control studies, for which the outcome variable is usually case status, with case = 1 and control = 0. For outcome variables that are other types of yes/no variables, it is typical to let yes = 1 and no = 0. Predictor variables for a logistic regression can be categorical or continuous.

The output for the regression model predicting being a case (not a control) is:

	β	SE	OR (95% CI)	p-value
sex	0.59	0.49	1.8 (0.7, 4.7)	0.23
ate_food	1.44	0.52	4.2 (1.5, 11.7)	0.01
constant	−0.82	0.37		0.03

OR for sex = exp(β) = exp(0.59) = 1.8

lower bound of 95%CI = exp(β − 1.96*SE) = exp(0.59 − 1.96*0.49) = 0.7

upper bound of 95%CI = exp(β + 1.96*SE) = exp(0.59 + 1.96*0.49) = 4.7

OR for ate_food = exp(β) = exp(1.44) = 4.2

lower bound of 95%CI = exp(β − 1.96*SE) = exp(1.44 − 1.96*0.52) = 1.5

upper bound of 95%CI = exp(β + 1.96*SE) = exp(1.44 + 1.96*0.52) = 11.7

Controlling for "ate_food" (a yes/no variable for whether participants ate a certain food), there is no difference by sex in the odds of being a case:
OR = 1.8 (0.7, 4.7)

Controlling for sex, those who ate the suspected food item had significantly higher odds of being a case than those who did not eat the item:
OR = 4.2 (1.5, 11.7)

The r^2 for the model is $r^2 = 0.14$, which means that the predictor variable explains 14% of the variation in the values of the outcome variable.

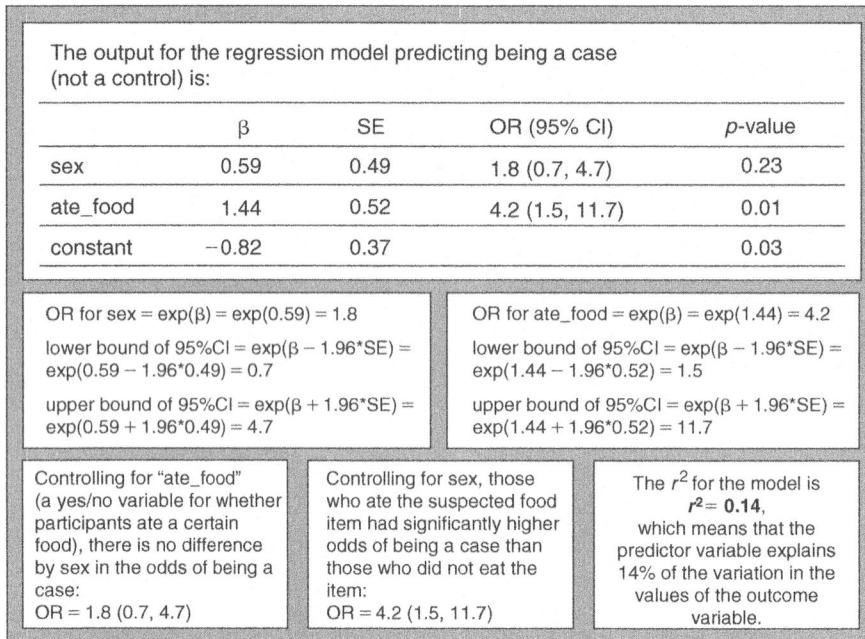

Note that 1.96 is used as a multiplier for a 95% confidence interval, 2.576 for a 99% CI, and 1.645 for a 90% CI.
FIGURE 28-7 Example of a Multiple Logistic Regression Model

FIGURE 28-7 provides an example of the output for a logistic regression and explains how to interpret it. The coefficient for a predictor variable in a logistic regression model is the natural log of the odds ratio, ln(OR). So the odds ratio for the association between that predictor variable and the outcome variable can be found by taking the exponential of the coefficient, $\exp(\beta)$. The odds ratio for each predictor variable represents the change in the odds of the outcome—typically the odds of being a case or being classified as a yes—for a 1-unit change in the predictor variable. The confidence interval for the odds ratio can be calculated using the value of the coefficient and its standard error, as shown in the figure.

■ 28.5 Dummy Variables

The predictor variables in regression models can take a variety of forms but must have numeric responses. Nominal categorical variables have responses that cannot be ordered and assigned a rank, but a series of *dummy variables* that convert categorical responses to a series of dichotomous (0/1) variables can be created. Additionally, when fitting a logistic regression model, it might be helpful to convert ratio and interval vari-

	Then the Values of the Dummy Variables Are . . .			
If the Response to the Original Question Was . . .	B_Dummy (Was B the response to the original question?)	C_Dummy (Was C the response to the original question?)	D_Dummy (Was D the response to the original question?)	Conclusion Based on the Dummy Variables
A	0 (no)	0	0	The response was not B, C, or D, so it was A.
B	1 (yes)	0	0	The response was B.
C	0	1	0	The response was C.
D	0	0	1	The response was D.

FIGURE 28-8 **Dummy Variables**

ables to dummy variables so that a series of odds ratios for the levels of the variable can be estimated.

FIGURE 28-8 provides an example of how this recoding works. If the original categorical variable has n possible responses, then $n - 1$ dummy variables are required to capture all the responses to the original question. All $n - 1$ variables should be included in a regression model (even if some may be eliminated during a stepwise selection process).

■ 28.6 Survival Analysis

Survival analysis examines the distribution of the durations of time that individuals in a study population experience from an initial time point (such as the time of enrollment in a study or the time of diagnosis of a particular condition) until some well-defined event, which can be death or some other outcome. Measures of survival include:

- Median survival time.
- Cumulative survival at set times after diagnosis.
- Life tables that record conditional and cumulative probabilities of survival.
- Kaplan-Meier plots that display cumulative survival rates (FIGURE 28-9).

Log-rank tests can be used to determine whether survival is shorter in one population than in another. Cox proportional hazards regression, which estimates a hazard ratio that compares durations to an event (such as death) in two populations, can also be used for survival analysis.

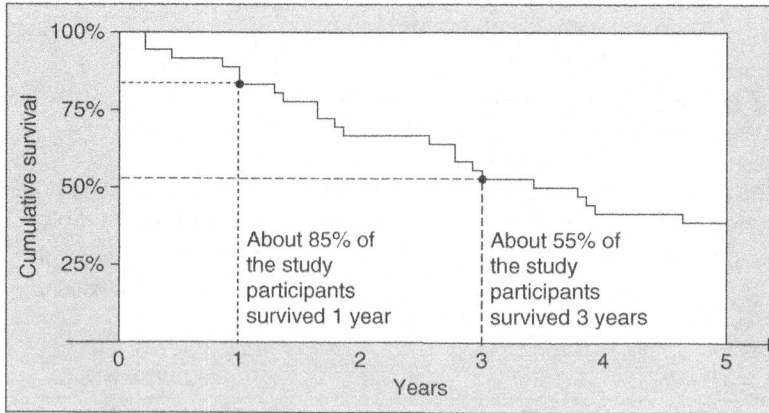

FIGURE 28-9 Example of a Kaplan-Meier Plot

■ 28.7 GIS/Spatial Analysis

If GPS (global positioning system) coordinates or other geographic data have been collected, then spatial software programs may be useful for conducting the geographic portion of the analysis. The geographic data should be incorporated into a *GIS (geographic information system)*. The GIS allows for spatial analysis such as:

- The identification of spatial disease clusters (using a statistic like Moran's coefficient or Geary's coefficient).
- The determination of associations, if any, between the social or physical environment and disease.
- The estimation of distances between locations.
- The ascertainment of the geographic factors that are related to access to health services.

A medical geography or health geography reference should be consulted for assistance with spatial analysis.

Reporting Findings

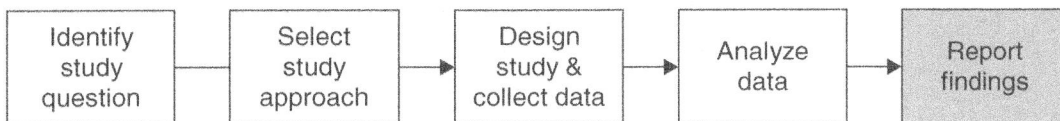

Identify study question	→	Select study approach	→	Design study & collect data	→	Analyze data	→	Report findings

The fifth and final step in the research process is to write a research report and prepare it for presentation and publication. This section provides tips for writing, revising, and disseminating findings.

- Article structure
- Citing
- Writing strategies
- Critically revising
- Posters and presentations
- Selecting target journals
- The submission, review, and publication process
- Why publish?

Article Structure

Research articles almost always have the same structure: abstract, introduction, methods, results, and discussion.

■ 29.1 Abstract

The *abstract* is a summary of the article. Its most important function is to serve as an advertisement for the manuscript because most computer databases and search engines have access only to abstracts. Even when researchers have a copy of the full text of an article, they will not be likely to read past the abstract if does not draw their attention. Therefore, an abstract ought to be accurate, reasonably complete, and compelling. Writing the abstract can be a challenge when most journals limit abstracts to a maximum of 150 to 250 words. It is usually easiest to write the abstract after the rest of the paper has already been written and the focus, key results, and conclusions are clear.

A *structured abstract* uses subheadings, like objective, methods, results, and conclusion, to highlight content.

An *unstructured abstract* usually follows the same outline but does not list the section titles.

■ 29.2 Introduction

The *introduction* provides the background information that a reader must know to understand the methods and results of the article. This section often includes information about the study population, the study site, and the study years. Person, place, and time characteristics are usually included somewhere in the text of the article in addition to appearing in the abstract.

The length of the introduction section compared to the discussion section varies according to the target publication venue. For some journals, a typical introduction might consist of only one or two paragraphs, but a lengthy discussion section is expected. For other journals, the introduction might be several pages long, but the discussion section is relatively short.

The introduction section might include a comparison to previous studies and a discussion of what is novel about the new study, but that content might appear in the discussion section instead. Some introductions provide a list of key definitions, but these might be placed in the methods section. No matter how much information is provided in the opening paragraphs of the paper, most introduction sections conclude with a statement about the importance or significance of the study and the specific aims, objectives, or hypotheses that the paper will address.

■ 29.3 Methods

The *methods* section should begin by clearly identifying the study design used. If person, place, and time characteristics were not provided in the introduction, they should be listed in this section. Definitions should be provided for the key exposures, outcomes, and other variables. For example, for a case-control study, the case definition should be spelled out; for an experimental study, the intervention and control should both be described in detail. For some studies, supplying the exact phrasing and order of questionnaire items, along with the steps taken to validate the survey instrument, might be important.

For primary studies, the methods used to identify, sample, and recruit participants should be described and the inclusion and exclusion criteria listed. The methods for collecting data should also be described, including interview techniques and (if relevant) laboratory methods and physical examination checklists and measurement methods. For secondary analyses, the report should specify who collected the data originally, how they were collected, how they were acquired for secondary analysis, and the role, if any, that the authors of the new paper had in data collection.

The methods section should provide information about ethical considerations, such as whether inducements were offered, how informed consent was documented, whether community groups were consulted, and which research ethics committees reviewed the project. Ethical issues can also be included in the endmatter, depending on the preference of the journal.

This section should end with a description of the statistical methods used.

The methods section can often be written even before data collection begins because most of the methods are finalized before data collection starts.

29.4 Results

The *results* section should start with a description of the study population that clearly identifies the sample size and the demographics of the participants. Additional results of statistical analysis should then be provided, using tables and figures when possible. Most studies do not require fancy multivariate statistics. The results of a statistical test should not be reported unless the authors fully understand when that test can be used and how it should be interpreted.

29.5 Discussion

The *discussion* section usually begins with a summary of the key findings of the new study. Ideally, the key findings should match the aims, objectives, or hypotheses spelled out in the last paragraph of the introduction section. The ensuing paragraphs should compare the new study to previous studies and include a thorough discussion of the relevant existing literature and an adequate number of citations.

Every paper needs to include at least one paragraph on the limitations of the study. The limitations paragraph should identify potential problems (such as types of bias) that could make the study results invalid or inaccurate. It should also explain the steps taken to minimize problems and why it is unlikely that serious problems occurred.

The final paragraph of the discussion should state the conclusions of the study. The appropriate conclusions vary by discipline and journal, but they might include new theories that emerge from the analysis, the policy implications of the study, or directions for future research.

29.6 Endmatter

Some journals list information between the conclusion and the reference list. The so-called *endmatter* may include:

- The affiliations of the authors and their contact information (if this is not listed on the title page)
- The contributions of each author to the paper

- Acknowledgments of people who assisted with the study but who did not meet authorship criteria
- Information about some ethical aspects of research (such as a declaration that each participant gave informed consent or the names and locations of the committees that reviewed the project)
- A list of all funding sources
- Disclosures of the presence or absence of possible conflicts of interest (both personal financial conflicts of interest and potential conflicts related to being employed by an organization with a financial interest in the study)

Some journals provide this information in the final published version of the paper but request that it be removed from the submitted manuscript. The reason is that some journals use a double-blind review process, and this information could reveal the identities or affiliations of the authors. Author guidelines of each journal will indicate what information should be provided in the endmatter.

■ 29.7 Tables and Figures

Many health journals limit the number of tables and figures allowed for each article, often to a maximum total of four (tables and figures combined). This limit means that the content for tables and figures must be carefully selected to highlight the most important aspects of the study. *Tables* should be used to organize and present statistical results that cannot easily be listed in the text in a sentence or two. Graphs and other *figures* should be used when a visual presentation of the material is more effective than words at conveying a result. Any images used should be meaningful, not merely decorative. There is no need to repeat information in the text that is provided in a table or figure, but be sure to have a *callout* for each table and figure that indicates when the reader should refer to the table or figure.

A table should provide enough information so that it can be independently interpreted and understood even in the absence of the text (FIGURE 29-1).

- The title of the table should provide a brief but clear description of the content.
- The rows and columns should each have a descriptive label and, when applicable, provide units and/or sample sizes (which are often designated by n for the number of participants).
- For each statistic, provide a confidence interval, p-value, and/or other measure of uncertainty, such as a standard deviation or standard error for a mean or an interquartile range for a median.
- A note just below the table (or in the title bar) should explain the meaning of asterisks (*) and other symbols (such as †, ‡, and §) commonly used to denote statistical significance and other items of interest.

Total Participants	*n*	87
Sex	*n* (%)	
Male		47 (54%)
Female		40 (46%)
Temperature at admission (°F)	Mean (SD)	100.3° (0.9°)
Symptoms at admission	*n* (%)	
Diarrhea		80 (92%)
Vomiting		56 (64%)
Cough		9 (10%)

FIGURE 29-1 Example Frequency Table for a Case Series

- Consistent fonts, spacing, and number of decimal points should be used for all tables in the manuscript.

A *graph* should provide enough information in the title, figure, and/or legend or key for a reader to be able to interpret the graph even without reading the related portion of the text. FIGURE 29-2 highlights some of the features that may make a graph easier or more difficult to interpret correctly.

High-resolution photographs, maps, flowcharts, and other images provided by the authors can also be used as figures. Note that photographs of study participants are usually not allowed without the written permission of the subject or subjects.

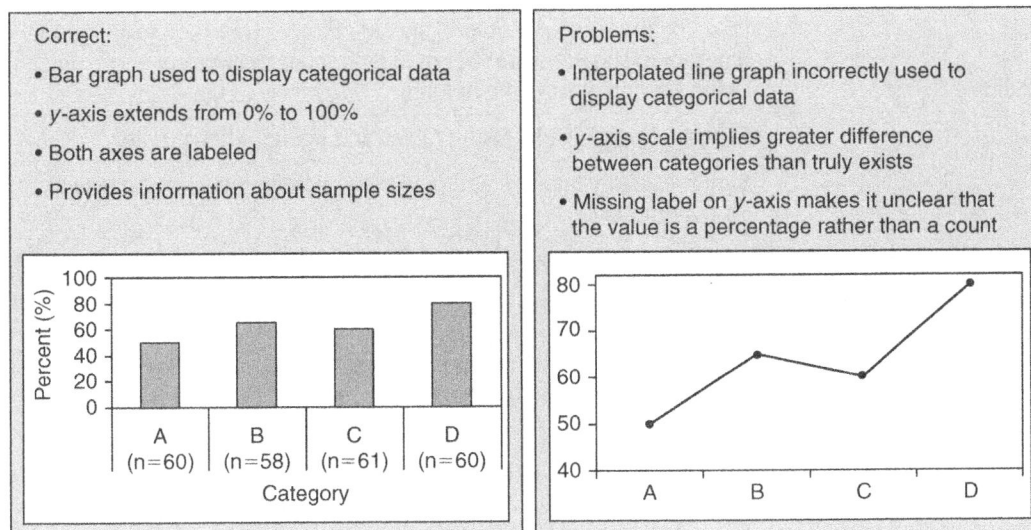

FIGURE 29-2 Examples of Correct and Problematic Graphs

■ 29.8 Writing Checklists

The most common information included in each section of an article is shown in FIG-URE 29-3.

Section	Content
Abstract/summary	Summarize the article using key words.
Introduction/background	Provide essential background information.
	State the objectives of the study (or, for experimental studies, the hypotheses tested).
Methods	Identify the study design (including, for experimental studies, the randomization method).
	Describe the source population (including selection methods and eligibility criteria and, if applicable, recruiting methods), the setting, and the dates of the study.
	Define key exposures, key outcomes, and other variables.
	Explain how data were collected.
	Describe how the required study size was estimated.
	Discuss ethical considerations (such as which research ethics committees approved the project, whether an inducement was offered, and how informed consent was documented).
	Describe the statistical methods used for analysis.
Results	Describe the study population, including the sample size (using a flow diagram to show the number of individual participants at each stage of the study if that will be helpful).
	Report relevant results (using tables and figures when possible).
Discussion	Summarize key findings and how they relate to the study objectives (or hypotheses).
	Discuss the limitations of the study.
	Provide a conservative and well-supported interpretation of the results, state how the new study fits with other relevant evidence (such as previous studies), and discuss the generalizability of the study (the populations to which findings might reasonably apply).
Endmatter	Acknowledge the contributions of each author, the assistance by people who did not meet authorship criteria (if any), the sources of funding, and potential conflicts of interest (if any), if requested by the journal.
	References.

FIGURE 29-3 Key Content for Articles Reporting on Analysis of Individual-Level Data

A number of checklists have been developed for the content to include in reports on various types of studies. Some of the most widely used checklists are listed in FIGURE 29-4.

Study Approach	Checklist	
Systematic review	PRISMA	Preferred Reporting Items for Systematic Reviews and Meta-Analyses (for evaluations of interventions)
Meta-analysis	PRISMA	
	MOOSE	Meta-analysis of Observational Studies in Epidemiology
Cross-sectional survey	STROBE—cross-sectional	Strengthening the Reporting of Observational Studies in Epidemiology
Case-control study	STROBE—case-control	
Cohort study	STROBE—cohort	
Experimental study	CONSORT	Consolidated Standards of Reporting Trials (for randomized controlled trials)
	TREND	Transparent Reporting of Evaluations with Nonrandomized Designs
Qualitative studies	COREQ	Consolidated Criteria for Reporting Qualitative Research

FIGURE 29-4 Common Reporting Guidelines

Citing

Research reports must provide accurate reference information for every publication that is used to support the methods, findings, and conclusions of a new study.

■ 30.1 Referring to the Scientific Literature

Authors of every new scientific paper need to explain how their new research fits with previous studies. The introduction section of a manuscript usually provides the background necessary to understand the importance of the new work. The discussion section typically provides an extensive comparison of the results of the new study to the results of previously published works. A typical article in the health sciences refers to about 20 or 30 other articles published in peer-reviewed journals, although some cite only a handful and some (especially review articles) may cite hundreds.

Pertinent articles can be found by searching electronic databases and by looking at the reference lists of articles already identified and determined to be helpful, since these sources are likely to also be related. (See Chapter 3 for a review of how to find relevant articles.) References should be carefully selected to support the importance, validity, and conclusions of the study. References can also be used to acknowledge the alternative methodological approaches that could have been used, to identify both areas in which the new findings agree with the existing literature and areas where the findings contradict previous studies, and to provide varying perspectives on the policy and practice implications of the study.

Citing an article is a way of endorsing the work of its authors (except in the rare instances when specific flaws need to be pointed out). So it is important to read the full text of every cited article and make sure that the methods and conclusions are sound. (Reading the full article carefully is even more important when criticizing the work.) Do not trust abstracts to be reliable. Abstracts may incorrectly or incompletely summarize the methods and results of a study. For example, they may leave out critical information, like a very small sample size, a very low participation rate, or the use of a data set that is many decades old. Or they may report only the statistics that are most shocking or the most congruent with previous studies. Additionally, abstracts often state conclusions that the study's data do not support. Before citing any article, read and understand the full article.

Journal articles are the preferred source of evidentiary support for scientific articles, although books, book chapters, and formal reports (such as those published by governmental agencies and international organizations) are also acceptable. FIGURE 30-1 summarizes the characteristics of formal reports, like those typically found in peer-reviewed journals. Fact sheets, websites, and other materials that have not been published in a formal online or print venue by a trusted organization should be cited only when a more reliable and permanent source of information is not available (FIGURE 30-2).

Formal Scientific Reports ...
Are published in a peer-reviewed journal (or sometimes a peer-reviewed report or book), not on a website, in a newspaper, or in a popular magazine.
Describe the study design and explain why it was appropriate for the objectives of the study.
Explain how the study population was selected and demonstrate that the sample size was sufficiently large.
Explain how exposures and outcomes were defined and assessed.
Describe the analytic approaches used and present results using easily interpreted tables and graphs.
Draw conclusions that are reasonable and based on the study's data.
Discuss the limitations of the study.
Compare the new study to previous studies.
Follow a standard outline and other conventions for scientific writing.

FIGURE 30-1 Characteristics of Formal Scientific Reports

Source	Formal or Informal?	Citable?	Remarks
Website or fact sheet	Informal	Rarely	Websites and fact sheets may be helpful starting places for informal research but should only be cited in a formal manuscript if they are from a trusted organization and no formal article or report provides the same information.
Newspaper or popular magazine	Informal	Rarely	Popular media items should be referred to only when no formal scientific article or report provides the same information.
Statistical database	Formal	Yes	Cite statistical databases and reports only if it is clear who collected the data, how it was collected, and when it was collected.
Official report	Formal	Yes	Reports are usually cited only when they are formal publications (with assigned publication years and/or other bibliographic information) from trusted organizations.
Book or book chapter	Formal	Yes	Although most scientific communication occurs through journals rather than books, scientific books are acceptable sources for formal manuscripts; general textbooks are rarely appropriate sources, but some highly technical textbooks are appropriate to cite.
Abstract	Formal	No	Cite only full-text articles (and be sure to read the full text before citing them).
Article	Formal	Yes	Articles from peer-reviewed journals are the preferred references for formal manuscripts.

FIGURE 30-2 **Citable Sources**

■ 30.2 Writing in One's Own Words

Few scientific articles quote directly from another source word for word. There are many reasons to avoid quoting from another publication. One of the most important is that borrowing phrases and sentences from other writers can make the writing in a document choppy. Some people who use quotes do so because they feel that the original works were so perfectly written that they could not say the same thing equally well using different words. This is not true. Saying the "same thing" in one's own writing style usually is better for the new work because it means that the entire article has the same voice.

Another benefit of paraphrasing is that it helps ensure that the article being cited has been understood. Paraphrasing accurately requires a level of comprehension that direct quoting does not. Using a quote that is not fully understood is never a good idea.

Paraphrasing does not remove the requirement to cite an original source; it just means that quotation marks do not have to be used. When a direct quote is lifted from a paper and reused, the entire quote must be in quotation marks (or indented from the left margin, depending on the length of the quote and journal formatting preferences). Additionally, an in-text citation must be provided. When the ideas or findings of other scholars are paraphrased, quotation marks are not used (because the words are not

Quotation (Almost Never Used in Journal Articles)	Paraphrase (Often Used)	Reference (Always Required for Either a Quotation or a Paraphrase)
A case-control study examining risk factors for ovarian cancer in Canadian women found that "age at first full-term pregnancy was not associated with risk of ovarian cancer."[1]	A case-control study of Canadian women found no association between ovarian cancer and the ages of participants at the time of their first full-term pregnancies.[1]	1. Risch HA, Marrett LD, Jain M, Howe GR. Differences in risk factors for epithelial ovarian cancer by histologic type: results of a case-control study. *Am J Epidemiol* 1996;144:363–72.
The authors acknowledged that "since we did not adjust for depth of inhalation and age at smoking onset, the RR for women, compared with that for men, due to smoking was likely to have been underestimated by our results."[2]	The authors of the study pointed out that it was possible that they might have underestimated the magnitude of the increased risk of lung cancer in female smokers compared to male smokers because they had not statistically adjusted for smoking behaviors, such as the depth of inhalation.[2]	2. Zang EA, Wynder EL. Differences in lung cancer risk between men and women: examination of the evidence. *J Natl Cancer Inst* 1996;88:183–92.
The investigators noted that "cholera is usually considered to be a water-borne disease, but, in this outbreak, the available evidence indicates that a food item served as part of a meal was the most likely vehicle of infection."[3]	The investigators concluded that the most likely cause of the cholera outbreak was food served to passengers on the airplane.[3]	3. Sutton RG. An outbreak of cholera in Australia due to food served in flight on an international aircraft. *J Hyg (London)* 1974;72:441–51.

FIGURE 30-3 Examples of Quoting and Paraphrasing

being copied), but an in-text citation for the source of the original information must still be provided. FIGURE 30-3 illustrates the difference between a quotation and a paraphrase.

■ 30.3 What Is Common Knowledge?

Any *specific knowledge*, such as a statistic or the results of a particular field or laboratory study, must be cited when it is referred to in a scientific paper. However, some areas of general knowledge, or common knowledge, do not require a citation. *Common knowledge* refers to what a typical person in the discipline would know; it does not refer to what a randomly selected person at the grocery store would know. For example, it would be common knowledge that influenza is caused by a virus and that Germany is located in Europe. Both of these facts are well established, and a quick search for papers on influenza or about studies conducted in Germany would show that this information is not usually accompanied by a citation. In contrast, a comment about the results of a particular epidemiological study of flu in Germany or a statistic about the proportion of Germans affected by flu in a typical year is specific knowledge; it would need to be cited. When in doubt about whether a bit of information is common knowledge, err on the side of using a citation. Also, any disputed fact should be well supported by one or more reliable sources.

■ 30.4 Avoiding Plagiarism

Plagiarism occurs when someone's wording, thinking, or creative output is repeated in a new document without attribution. Copying the exact words of another person without using quotation marks and providing a full citation, paraphrasing a unique theory or observation without providing a citation, and using an image without permission and an acknowledgment are all forms of plagiarism. Failing to acknowledge the source of the original work deprives the author or creator of the material the recognition that the person deserves, and it may result in the plagiarist getting credit for work that he or she did not do.

Plagiarism is a major violation of scholarly integrity, and it can have a damaging long-term impact on a professional career. For example, a published article with extensive plagiarism must be retracted, which requires the public acknowledgment of guilt and results in a permanent open record of wrongdoing. (The consequences of plagiarism and other forms of research misconduct, such as redundant publication or the fabrication or falsification of data, are discussed in detail on the website of the Committee on Publication Ethics.) For students, plagiarism can result in expulsion from school.

Several habits can be adopted to ensure that plagiarism does not occur. One helpful practice is never to cut and paste information from a website, article, or any other source into a document file that contains any draft material for an article. It is far too easy for those words, phrases, or even whole sentences to be unintentionally incorporated into the text of a manuscript. When browsing websites for background material, take the time to paraphrase the information rather than cutting and pasting the content for later review.

Another good habit is always to include a reference in research notes about any observation that will later require a citation. For example, if an article presents a theory that explains the findings of the new project, do not just make a note about the theory. Jot it down and put a bracket with the author and year next to it, as in a journal manuscript. Also write out the full bibliographic information for the article so that the source of the theory can be easily identified later on when writing is under way.

■ 30.5 Citation Styles

Citations typically appear in two formats:

- As in-text citations where the sources of information are briefly identified in the text.
- In a reference list at the end of the document that provides full bibliographic information for each source.

No one citation style is used in the health sciences. Most medical and public health journals use some version of a style alternately called ICMJE (International Committee of Medical Journal Editors) style or Vancouver style, or they use the very similar NLM (National Library of Medicine) style or AMA (American Medical Association) style. Alternately, a journal may adopt the APA (American Psychological Association) style or some other style. (APA style is commonly used for social science journals as well as for nursing journals.) However, although some journals strictly adhere to one widely used reference style, many have their own customized styles. Reference manuals and style guides are available for all of the widely used styles, and most journals provide an author's guide on their websites that spells out the journal's own style. Articles recently published in the target journal provide additional examples of the journal's preferred style. Whether preparing a manuscript for publication or writing a less formal report, the goal should be to use a consistent citation and reference style throughout the document.

In-text citations are abbreviated bits of information about the cited work that allow the full reference to be located in the reference list at the end of the article. Examples of formats for in-text citations are shown in FIGURE 30-4. (Some journals will convert bracketed citations to superscript numbers during the editing and layout process. The author guidelines must be carefully examined to see which submission style is preferred.)

Number of Citations for the Sentence	1 Source	2 Sources	3 Sources
First author's last name and publication year	… (Ruiz, 2004).	… (Ruiz, 2004; Yamamoto, 2001).	… (Ivanov, 2008; Ruiz, 2004; Yamamoto, 2001).
Author(s) and publication year	… (Ruiz, 2004).	… (Ruiz & Sanchez, 2004; Yamamoto et al., 2001).	… (Ivanov, 2008; Ruiz & Sanchez, 2004; Yamamoto et al., 2001).
Number in brackets (square brackets)	… [1].	… [1, 2].	… [1−3].
	… .[1]	… .[1, 2]	… .[1−3]
Number in parentheses (round brackets)	… (1).	… (1,2).	… (1−3).
	… .(1)	… .(1,2)	… .(1−3)
Superscript number	… .[1]	… .[1,2]	… .[1−3]

FIGURE 30-4 In-Text Citation Styles

The reference list at the end of the article presents cited works either alphabetically by the first author's last name or in the order of first appearance of the cited work in the text of the article. When preparing a manuscript for submission to a journal, check the document carefully for compliance with the journal's house style. Journals that use ICMJE style or a variant typically list authors by last name and first initials, then the title (with capital letters only for proper nouns), an abbreviated journal name, the publication year, volume, and page numbers. The components may be separated by periods (full stops) or by semicolons or commas. However, the journals may make minor adjustments to these components. Some journals expect all authors to be listed no matter how many there are; some journals use an abbreviated version for six or more authors, such as listing only the first three authors, followed by "et al." Some use abbreviations for journals; others use the full journal name. Some list issue numbers; most do not. Some list the full page numbers (such as 202–209), and others use a slightly shorter version (such as 202–9). Some use italics or bold type for some parts of the bibliographic entry. The key is to be consistent, no matter which style is adopted.

Writing Strategies

This chapter provides tips for moving through the writing process successfully.

■ 31.1 The Writing Process

By the time a researcher is ready to write a final report about a project, the vast majority of the work on the project has been completed: A study question has been identified and refined, a study approach has been selected and a protocol developed, and data have been collected and analyzed. The end of the project is in sight, but the prospect of creating a report that is intended to be disseminated beyond those immediately involved in the project can be intimidating. Putting off the writing process is easy. The writing can drag on, and in some cases it is never completed.

Few writers have the ability to sit down and crank out a complete manuscript in one burst of productivity. Most writers experience cycles of high motivation and productivity and then of absolutely no interest in their work. So most writers have to find strategies to get the first words on paper and then to see the manuscript through to completion. FIGURE 31-1 illustrates a typical writer's productivity levels during the writing process. The durations of each stage will vary among writers and for different papers, but writers usually need to address their motivation at three key times.

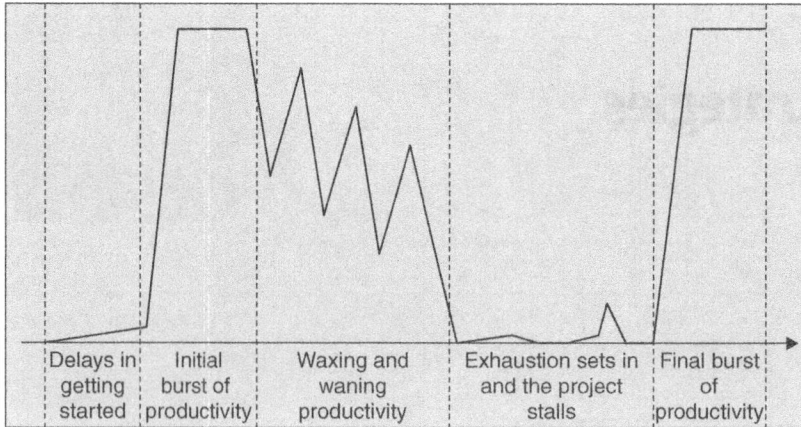

FIGURE 31-1 Typical Variations in Productivity during the Writing Process

- First, writers must overcome the barriers to getting started.
- Second, writers must find ways to prolong the period of high productivity that often occurs at the start of a writing project.
- Finally, most writers become fatigued during the writing process and at some point lose all desire even to think about their projects. At such points, they must find the motivation to persevere and to complete the manuscript.

■ 31.2 Getting Started

Scientific papers follow a standard outline (see Chapter 29). There is no need to think creatively about the structure of a paper. By the time a researcher has defined a study question, designed a study, collected data, and analyzed data, there should be sufficient information to answer the key study question and explain the findings. At that point, the only way to get started on a writing project is to start writing.

If a researcher does not know how to begin writing, an easy way to start filling pages is to:

- Put a working title for the paper at the beginning of the file, along with the names of all the coauthors.
- Add in the headers for the Abstract, Introduction, Methods, Results, Discussion, Acknowledgments, and References.
- Fill in the names of the people to thank in the acknowledgments section.
- Add page numbers.
- Paste in a table or figure that was created during the analysis process and will be included in the final report.
- Paste in some relevant lines about methods from the protocol.

Then start filling in the gaps. Perhaps find a model article and use it as a template to create a detailed outline that specifies exactly what each paragraph in the paper will cover. For example, the headers for paragraphs on statistical methods and ethical considerations can be inserted at the end of the methods section. A brief list of what to cover in each of those paragraphs can then be added based on what was reported in the model article. (Be careful not to plagiarize any ideas or phrases from the model article.) Then write a sentence or two for each of those key points: a sentence about informed consent, a sentence about ethics committee review, a sentence about the significance level used for statistical tests.

The content of the manuscript does not need to be added in any particular order. Many authors of scientific papers find it easiest to start with the methods, then to write the results, then the introduction and discussion, and finally the abstract, but that order is not required. Many authors skip around in the paper, adding a few sentences at a time here and there. Some authors find it helpful to write throughout the research process. They may draft the introduction as soon as the study question has been identified, the methods once the study is designed, and the results after data have been collected and analyzed. Then they draft the discussion section and edit the earlier drafts of the manuscript to ensure that the paper tells a focused story. When getting started, a good plan is to first write whatever part of the paper is ready to be put into words. Then just keep on writing.

■ 31.3 Staying Motivated

Most writers experience times when they have no desire at all to write. A number of steps can help a writer to regain motivation. Sometimes changing habits or scenery helps—writing in a new place or at a new time of day or removing distractions from the writing area. Sometimes setting a time line for completing small parts of the paper is helpful. A time line makes it easier to see tasks being accomplished. Build in rewards that celebrate those intermediate successes on the way to a completed paper.

Many manuscripts for health science journals are limited to a maximum of about 3000 words. So writing only 100 words a day—just a few sentences—will lead to a completed first draft of a manuscript in less than two months. Revising the paper may take another month or two of daily writing (see Chapter 32). Time lines and goals can be set for that process as well.

Setting up a weekly meeting with an advisor or a writing group may also help with staying on track. If the mental block is truly about the content of the manuscript, talking through the project with a friend can be helpful. Another approach is to speak the content aloud or write it very informally or in sentence fragments. The ideas that emerge from these exercises can be formalized later. Alternatively, move on to a different section while waiting for inspiration about the trickier parts of the paper.

■ 31.4 Conquering Writer's Block

Sometimes a case of *writer's block* gets serious and can last for weeks or months. FIGURE 31-2 lists various types of writer's block. In each case, a negative thought cycle develops that has to be broken. Acknowledging the underlying issues—fear of being judged and fear of failure are common—is one step toward getting back to writing. But writers also need to initiate new behaviors to facilitate success.

One remedy is to set aside something like 30 minutes at the same time each day for writing. Then stay at a desk with a writing tablet or a word processor for the full 30 minutes with no distractions: no videos, no music, no computer games, no e-mail. Although it may take several days or even weeks for this dedicated writing time to result in meaningful output, writer's block can be overcome only when an aspiring writer makes writing time a priority. Additionally, those with writer's block benefit from consultations with senior coauthors, a writing support group, friends, and others who can help motivate them.

The completed manuscript will not be perfect. No paper is perfect. By the time a report is written, there are likely to be a lot of imperfections that cannot be fixed. For example, the methods used to select participants cannot be changed. Participants cannot be asked a question that was not included in the questionnaire. These flaws are normal and expected. What authors can do is:

- Fully explain the actual methods used
- Run all the appropriate analyses
- Include a helpful set of references that support the results
- Polish the prose
- Honestly identify the limitations of the study and explain what was done to address them

Reason to Avoid Writing	Reality Check
"This study is boring and unimportant."	Most studies make only minor contributions to moving a field forward, but the only way to make any contribution is to publish.
"This research project had some serious flaws: The premise was bad, the study design was poor, and the data collection didn't go perfectly."	Every study has flaws, but few are fatally flawed. Coauthors and/or advisors would not allow major mistakes to be made.
"I don't know how to write a scholarly paper."	The best way to learn how to write is by writing. A writing support group, coauthors, and/or advisors can help with this process.
"I'm stuck on this one section, and I can't work on anything else until I finish this part."	Writing and rewriting the same section over again or spending weeks searching the literature for more supporting evidence are both stall tactics. The best way to move forward is to work on another section of the paper or to ask a coauthor or advisor for assistance.
"I don't know what to do next."	Coauthors and/or advisors will be happy to offer advice about how to move forward.
"I don't want to disappoint/be criticized by my professor/supervisor."	Supervisors want a paper to be as good as it can be, and they are obligated to make suggestions about critical revisions if they are coauthors. A writing support group and/or a supportive, encouraging, and honest friend and/or colleague can review drafts before the manuscript is shared with a supervisor. Procrastination will only increase anxiety about being evaluated.
"I'm not a good writer." "I'm not good at writing in English."	Coauthors, advisors, and friends and/or colleagues can help polish the manuscript, but only after it has been drafted.
"I don't think this project was interesting enough to publish anything about it."	Check with a coauthor and/or advisor about how to appropriately disseminate the findings.
"If I submit this paper and it is rejected, I will be embarrassed."	Comments about a paper are not criticisms of a person. The only people who will know about the status of a manuscript are those whom the authors tell about it. Also, supervisors will know that many papers are submitted to several journals before they are accepted for publication. Procrastination will only delay the start of the review process and the possibility of acceptance and publication.
"If this paper is published, someone might discover a flaw in it, and that would be embarrassing."	Coauthors, reviewers, and editors will not let an obviously flawed or badly written article proceed to publication.
"I don't have time to write."	Almost everyone can find 15 or 30 minutes a day to write. Do not use "busyness" as an excuse to avoid writing.

FIGURE 31-2 Forms of Writer's Block

Critically Revising

Once a complete manuscript has been drafted, it needs to be revised and polished. Coauthors and other colleagues may help with this process, but the lead author is responsible for checking the manuscript very carefully. Three checklists are provided to facilitate the revision process.

■ 32.1 Does the Paper Have a "Plot"?

Every paper should tell a "story" that has:

- A beginning—the introduction sets the stage.
- A middle—the methods and results say what happened.
- An end—the discussion provides a conclusion that ties all the parts of the story together.

The story line should be able to be summarized in a sentence or two. Indeed, some journals require a *précis* that is 35 words or less. The abstract for the report should tell the whole story in one compelling paragraph. And the whole manuscript must also work to convey a cohesive message (FIGURE 32-1). The first step in editing is to make sure that the big picture is being clearly communicated.

Does the paper have a clear "story line"? Can the "plot" be summarized in one sentence?
Does the title of the paper reflect the key aspects of the study?
Does the abstract tell the key parts of the story?
Do the opening paragraphs draw the reader into the story?
Is the goal of the study clearly stated in the introduction section?
Does the methods section make it clear how the methods were helpful in answering the study question?
Do the results and discussion sections provide the answer to the study question?
Is the story missing any parts that need to be added so that it is complete and compelling? Do any gaps in logic need to be addressed?
Are any parts of the manuscript redundant? Are any parts peripheral to the main story? Can these be removed to tighten the story line?
Are the conclusions fully supported by the data?
Does each paragraph have a theme?

FIGURE 32-1 Does the Paper Tell a Compelling "Story"?

■ 32.2 Structure and Content

Once the pieces of the paper's story are clear, the next step is to check the structure and content of the manuscript (FIGURE 32-2). The paper should be well organized, complete but concise, and accurate about what was done and what was found. The text, the tables and figures, and the reference list must all meet these same requirements.

Is the paper well organized? Is the content focused?
Does the introduction provide all essential background information? (For example, are the person, place, and time details listed somewhere in both the abstract and the text?)
Does the introduction make the research project appear necessary and important?
Does the introduction say why the study is novel?
Are the methods described in adequate detail?
Is enough statistical analysis presented? Is each statistic included in the paper necessary?
Are the tables and figures well designed?

FIGURE 32-2 Checklist for the Structure and Content of the Paper

Are all statistics presented either in the figures or tables or in the text, but not in both?
Does the discussion provide a concise summary of key findings and then place the new findings in the context of previous research? Does the discussion section avoid simply reiterating the results section?
Does the discussion adequately address the potential limitations of the study?
Is every claim in the discussion section supported by citations? Should additional references be added to further support the key message of the paper?
Is every reference listed important and necessary? Can any entries in the reference list be cut?
Has the paper been double-checked to ensure that no part of it is plagiarized or paraphrased without proper attribution?
Is every part of the paper truthful? (For example, does the paper report the methods that were actually used rather than an idealized version of them? Does it report the results of the most appropriate statistical tests rather than results from less appropriate tests that happened to produce statistically significant results?)

FIGURE 32-2 (continued)

■ 32.3 Style and Clarity

In a final check, look at each word, sentence, paragraph, and section, examining style and clarity (FIGURE 32-3):

- Words must be used carefully.
- Sentences must be concise and clear.
- The voice must be consistent.
- The grammar and spelling must be proper throughout.

Are words used precisely? (For example, are terms like "associated," "correlated," and "caused" used appropriately? Are "incidence" and "prevalence" used correctly?)
Is unnecessary jargon avoided? Are definitions provided for all key terms?
Are all abbreviations introduced at first use?
Is the tone of the writing appropriate? Is the writing style fact based rather than emotion based?
Does the article consistently use a third-person voice or, in rare situations, consistently use a first-person ("I" or "we") voice? Is the voice correct for the target journals, if applicable?

FIGURE 32-3 Checklist for Style and Clarity

Do all subjects (nouns) agree with their associated verbs? (For example, since "data" is a plural word, is "data are …" used rather than "data is …"?) Are all other grammatical conventions followed?
Are active verbs rather than passive verbs used whenever possible?
Is the verb tense consistent? (For most papers the past tense is used rather than the present because the data were collected in the past.)
Is each sentence clear? Are phrases as concise as possible?
Are all words spelled correctly? (Each report should consistently follow the spelling conventions of one country.)
Is all punctuation correct? (For example, are there extra or missing commas?)
Does the paper adhere to the specifications of the target journal (if the manuscript is being prepared for submission to a journal)?

FIGURE 32-3 (continued)

Posters and Presentations

Research results are often publicly shared for the first time during an oral presentation or poster session at an academic or professional conference.

■ 33.1 Purpose of Conferences

The primary outcome of most professional and academic conferences is networking: meeting new people working in the same field of interest, catching up with old friends, and making and nurturing professional connections that may be helpful in the future. Conferences are a place to exchange ideas: to learn about what others in the field are doing, to learn new methods and techniques in a discipline, and to share current work with others and receive feedback on it. Presenting new research in the form of a poster or an oral presentation can be a particularly useful way to get feedback on a project before submitting the work for review by a journal. Sharing findings is a way to gauge what others find most interesting about the project and to identify the weaker aspects of the study and the questions that need to be addressed in a formal written manuscript.

■ 33.2 Structure of Conferences

Some conferences are annual events sponsored by professional organizations that draw thousands of attendees. Others are small gatherings of a few dozen scholars working in a narrow field of study. Most conferences include a mix of:

- Plenary sessions where keynote addresses are given
- Business meetings run by the officers of the sponsoring organization
- Concurrent sessions in which multiple panels of oral presentations are held at the same time in different rooms
- Poster sessions in which attendees can mingle while reviewing research posters

Presenters are usually assigned to deliver either an oral presentation or a poster presentation. *Oral presentations* require speaking in front of a potentially large audience and may involve facing an open question-and-answer period in which the work can be discussed. This interaction can be helpful in improving the work prior to publication—so much so that some presenters are disappointed when no one in the audience raises a concern about their work. However, the process can be incredibly stressful. Oral presentations are generally considered to be more prestigious than posters, in part because there are usually more slots for poster presenters than for oral presenters.

Poster sessions are usually held in a less formal venue. Posters may be taped along the walls of a room or displayed on long rows of easels, and attendees can browse through them at their own pace and interact with presenters if they want more information about a project. Having one-on-one or small group conversations about one's work can be very helpful. However, posters often require more preparation time than oral presentations, and they may also be expensive to print and a hassle to transport. (They are, however, nice to display in the hallway of an academic department or workplace for several months after the conference.)

■ 33.3 Submitting an Abstract

Researchers interested in presenting at a conference are usually required to submit an abstract for consideration by the organizing committee. The conference organizing committee and other reviewers:

- Rate the submitted abstracts.
- Decide which researchers will be invited to present.
- Select who will give an oral presentation as part of a panel and who will be assigned to a poster session.

Abstracts selected for a conference are usually printed in a conference bulletin for easy reference by attendees, to help them decide which sessions to attend and which posters to seek out.

A good abstract includes key words and conveys one clear health message that is appropriate to the audience expected at the conference. If the conference focuses on clinical practice, the abstract's applied message should be readily translatable into improved patient care. If the conference focuses on research theories and methods, the abstract should emphasize the novelty of the approaches used and their applicability to other research topics. If the conference focuses on health policy, the abstract should have a clear policy implication.

Since the submission deadline is often many months before the conference, somewhat preliminary results may need to be presented in the abstract. However, the objectives and methods must be clear, and, very importantly, final results must be ready to share by the conference dates.

Applicants may be asked about their preferred presentation formats. Those who indicate a willingness to do either an oral presentation or a poster may increase the likelihood that their abstracts will be accepted for the conference.

Submitting an abstract for consideration infers a commitment to attend the conference if selected to be a presenter. The fine-print instructions for the conference often specify the expectations of applicants. For example, the sponsoring organization may keep track of dropouts and absentees and not allow them to present at future conferences. Most conferences require presenters to pay a registration fee (often several hundred dollars) as well as cover all of their own travel expenses, although some schools and employers may reimburse some or all of these expenses.

■ 33.4 Preparing a Poster

Conference attendees are drawn to visually appealing posters. So when preparing a poster, give equal attention to its content and to its design (FIGURE 33-1). Posters should be

Content	Keep the content focused on one core message.
	Choose a descriptive title.
	Include author names, brief author affiliations, and contact information for at least one author.
	Do not list information about the conference (such as name, dates, or location) on the poster.
	Consider skipping the abstract to save space.
	Clearly state the main goal, the specific objectives or hypotheses, and the importance of the study.
	Use a structured format, with introduction/background, methods, results, and conclusion/discussion sections (and a reference list, in small font, if previous studies are cited).
	Be concise. Use short sentences and bulleted lists when possible.
	Images like graphs, tables, flowcharts, photographs, and maps are more effective than words at conveying information.

FIGURE 33-1 Suggestions for Poster Content, Layout, and Formatting

Layout and formatting	Find out the size and shape (horizontal or vertical) of the display area that the conference organizers will provide and create a poster to fill the space.
	Decide whether to print one large poster (preferred) or smaller panels that can be joined together at the conference venue.
	Organize content into three or four columns or another structure with a logical flow.
	Use boxes, color, and/or lines to group the information.
	Leave adequate white space, and keep the color palette simple.
	Ensure adequate contrast between the background (usually light) and content (usually dark). It is often helpful to use borders for photographs and other image content.
	Use large and consistent fonts that can easily be read several steps back from the poster.
	Simplify graphs and make sure that they can be read from a distance (which may require adding a title and directly labeling lines or bars rather than using a key).
	Use high-resolution images (and remember that enlarged photographs become fuzzy).

FIGURE 33-1 (continued)

well organized and have focused content, an eye-pleasing balance between text and images and white space, and an inviting color palette.

Posters can be created using either specialized graphic design software or a simple presentation software program like PowerPoint. The size of a slide can be adjusted so that the dimensions match those required by the conference. A sample layout is shown in FIGURE 33-2, and the Internet has many examples of other poster formats. Be sure to have several people check both the content and the design of the poster before it is printed. Also, inquire about:

- Printing costs (which will vary significantly depending on the size of the poster, the amount of color, the type of paper or fabric, and any special options like laminating or mounting)
- The amount of time required for printing
- Whether a special carrying case is needed

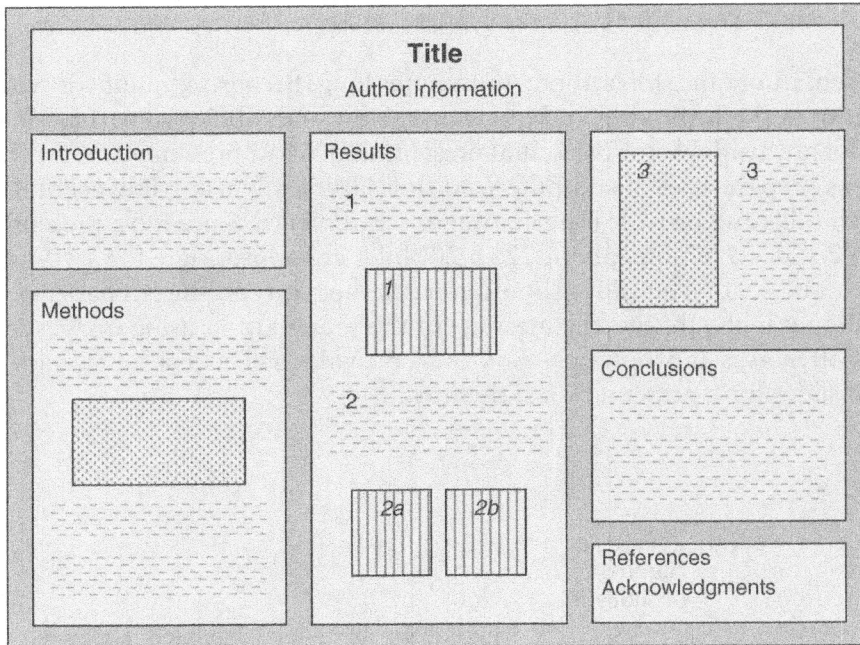

FIGURE 33-2 **Sample Poster Layout**

■ 33.5 Presenting a Poster

At most conferences, the poster presenter is responsible for setting up the poster at an assigned time. Although some conference organizers provide all the necessary supplies, presenters usually find out what is required only after they arrive at the conference site. Poster presenters should therefore come prepared with clips (for clipping a poster to a board set on an easel), pushpins (for pinning a poster to a corkboard), and tape (for taping a poster to a wall). The presenter is also responsible for taking down the poster at an appointed time. It is considered bad form to take down a poster early or to leave it up after the assigned time, when someone else may be waiting to set up a poster for the next session.

Some conferences designate poster session times when presenters are expected to stand by their posters and interact with attendees. These sessions are an opportunity for one-on-one conversations with interested individuals. It is appropriate to greet each person who stops to view the poster. Thus, the presenter should respond to questions without becoming so engaged with one person that all others with questions or comments are ignored. Some presenters prepare a handout that is either a page-sized printout of the full poster or a sheet with highlights. Most presenters have business cards with contact information available for distribution.

■ 33.6 Preparing for an Oral Presentation

A typical oral presentation time slot is about 15 minutes long. Because a minute or two is required for setup at the beginning and questions at the end, about 10 to 12 minutes of this time slot are available for the actual presentation. Most presenters at health science conferences prepare a set of computerized slides (typically using PowerPoint) that will guide their talks and provide information to the audience. Since most presenters can cover 1 or 2 slides a minute, about 12 to 20 slides are appropriate for a 10- to 12-minute talk (FIGURE 33-3). The slides should not attempt to reproduce a paper on the screen; they should highlight the key message of the presentation using images in place of words as often as is appropriate. FIGURE 33-4 provides a checklist for the content and layout of slides for a presentation slide show.

Content Area	Number of Slides	Note
Title slide	1	Include the title, names of authors, and contact information for the presenter.
Research goal/importance	1	Start with the key message.
Outline or summary	1	
Background/specific aims	1–2	Include citations (in small font) for any previous work mentioned and for images taken from other sources.
Methods	2–4	
Results	4–8	Figures and tables of statistical results usually need to be very simple to be readable during a presentation.
Strengths/limitations	1	
Conclusions	1	End with the key message.
Acknowledgments and/or invitation for questions	0–1	
Total	12–20	

FIGURE 33-3 Sample Distribution of Slides for a 10- to 12-Minute Talk

Content	Each slide has a title.
	The content of each slide is accurate.
	Graphs, tables, photographs, and other images are used in place of words as often as is appropriate.
	Key words and phrases are used instead of full sentences.
	There are no more than about six lines per slide.
	All words are spelled correctly.
	All phrases are grammatically correct.
	All bulleted phrases on one slide use a consistent voice (for example, all start with the word "to" or all start with an "-ing" word).
	The number of slides is appropriate for the scheduled presentation duration (about 1–2 slides per minute, excluding time set aside for questions).
	Every slide is relevant.
	The slides are in a logical order.
Layout and formatting	The background is simple and not distracting.
	There is an adequate contrast between the background and the text (either dark letters on a light background or light letters on a dark background). The contrast is adequate under different lighting conditions (for example, whether overhead lights are on or off).
	A consistent and readable font is used throughout.
	A large font size is used throughout, including tables and figures (which may require simplifying them and enlarging the font used for various components).
	A consistent and pleasant color scheme is used throughout.
	The slides are not cluttered.
	All tables and figures are readable.
	Unnecessary effects like sounds, animated components, and distracting slide transitions are avoided.

FIGURE 33-4 Checklist for Presentation Slide Show

Preparing the slide show is only the first step in preparing to make an oral presentation. FIGURE 33-5 provides a list of content-, voice-, and performance-related items to practice extensively in the weeks before a presentation. Practice in front of people who will provide honest feedback. Consider video-recording a practice performance, reviewing it, and identifying areas for improvement. No one can plan for everything that might be encountered at the conference, including nerves, but practice makes a positive experience more likely.

Content	Opening lines	Practice the exact opening sentences; these need to capture the attention of the audience.
	Message	Master the content of each slide enough to describe each one without referring to notes.
	Phrasing	Use relatively short, precise sentences with active verbs.
	Flow	Practice transitions from one slide to the next.
	Closing lines	Practice exact closing sentences about key conclusions.
Voice	Pace	Speak at a moderate to slow rate.
	Volume	Speak relatively loudly.
	Pitch	Vary your voice inflection.
	Enunciation	Speak clearly; avoid words and phrases that are difficult to pronounce, if possible.
	Pronunciation	Check on the pronunciation of technical words and names.
	Fillers	Try to avoid fillers (such as "um, . . . ah, . . . like . . . you know").
Performance	Engagement	Smile and make eye contact with members of the audience.
	Posture	Stand tall or sit straight.
	Delivery	Do not just read the slides or read from a script.
	Movement	Try not to fidget, sway, pace, or make other distracting gestures or movements.
	Technology	Become comfortable with advancing slides (using a mouse, keyboard, and/or clicker) and with using a pointer, if applicable; face the audience when using these tools, if possible.

FIGURE 33-5 Things to Practice Before the Presentation

A few weeks before the conference, confirm what equipment will be provided in the presentation room (such as a computer and an LCD projector).

- Some conferences expect presenters to provide their own laptop computers.
- Some conferences require presenters to upload their presentation files to a website in advance of the conference.
- Some ask presenters to e-mail their files to the session moderator.
- Some expect presenters to have the file on CD, and others prefer presentation files to be on a flash drive.

No matter what format is preferred, always bring a backup copy of the presentation file.

33.7 Giving an Oral Presentation

FIGURE 33-6 summarizes the key tasks on the day of the presentation. Conference organizers often advise presenters to:

- Arrive at the presentation room at least 15 minutes before the panel begins (not 15 minutes before an individual presentation time).
- Check in with the moderator.
- Set up the computer and projector or confirm that slides are ready to be projected.

Presenters are also often reminded to be considerate of other presenters in their session by strictly adhering to their assigned time limits.

At most conferences, time is allotted for questions from the audience, either after each presentation or after all the panelists in the session have spoken. If a microphone is not available for those asking questions, the respondent should repeat the question before answering it. The appropriate etiquette is usually to:

- Keep responses short.
- Thank those who offer suggestions for improving the work.
- Acknowledge the limitations of a study yet highlight its strengths.
- Be respectful to everyone.

At the end of the session, one-on-one or small group conversation about the research may continue. Presenters should have business cards available to give to those who have overlapping interests.

Time	Tasks	
15 minutes before the assigned presentation panel is scheduled to begin	Moderator	Check in with the session moderator or chair, if there is one.
	Q&A	Ask the moderator whether the question-and-answer time will take place after each presenter or after all the presenters are finished.
	Time	Confirm the amount of time for the presentation, and ask the moderator whether there is a timekeeper and what sort of warning signs will be given when the allotted time is nearly finished. If there is no timekeeper, ask a friendly person in the front row to serve as one.
	Computer	If using a computer and/or projector, check to be sure that the devices are set up and that the presentation is loaded on the computer and ready to use.
	Pointer	If using a pointer and/or clicker, check to be sure that they are working.
	Microphone	If using a microphone, check to be sure that it works.
	Water	Check to be sure that drinking water is available.
	Copresenters	Greet other presenters in the session.
During other presenters' talks in the session	Listen	Pay attention to the other talks; do not focus on personal notes or preparation during this time.
	Connect	Listen for points of connection between the research talks being presented, especially if the question-and-answer period comes at the end of the session.
During the talk	Relax	Trust that practice will result in a proficient presentation.
	Control	Be alert to nervous behaviors, such as adding fillers to speech or swaying the body.
	Keep time	Do not exceed the allotted time period.
After the talk	Thanks	Thank the moderator, timekeeper, technology support person, and/or fellow presenters.
	Belongings	Check to be sure that personal items are not forgotten.
	Conversations	Wait in the room for at least a few minutes in case anyone has follow-up questions; move the discussion into the hallway as soon as the presenters for the next session begin setting up their talks.

FIGURE 33-6 Checklist of Tasks on the Day of the Presentation

Selecting Target Journals

The culmination of a well-designed and carefully conducted health research project is often the dissemination of results through an appropriate publication.

■ 34.1 Choosing a Target Journal

Researchers who want to publish their findings must identify one or more journals that could reasonably be expected to disseminate their reports. Selecting a *target journal* early in the writing process makes it easier to hone the paper's message for the journal's audience. An examination of recent articles published in the target journal provides guidance about:

- The best outline to follow
- How to divide commentary between the introduction and discussion sections
- What subsections to include in the methods section
- The appropriate voice and writing style
- The amount of technical detail to include
- The reference and citation style

Choosing a target journal entails many considerations, including:

- The aim and scope of the journal
- Its audience
- Its impact factor and other characteristics
- The possible costs of publication
- Online access options

■ 34.2 Aim, Scope, and Audience

The most important considerations when considering potential target journals are the fit of the research topic with the aims, scope, and audience of the journal. Some journals are very broad in focus, while others are very narrow and publish in only one subspecialty area. Some are international journals that publish research from around the world. Others have a very specific local or regional focus and publish articles pertinent only to that geographic area.

Determining whether an article is a fit with a specialty or regional journal is often straightforward. As an example, a journal focused on liver disease in Argentina will not be interested in a paper about osteoporosis in Mongolia, but it will review a manuscript on cirrhosis in Buenos Aires. A journal focused on nutrition in Southeast Asia would not review a manuscript on vision disorders in Sweden, but it would consider a paper on iodine deficiency in Cambodia.

Knowing what topics fall within the scope of a general journal is a little harder. Some prestigious general journals will publish only articles expected to have a significant and nearly immediate impact on clinical practice. Some general journals in medicine, public health, nursing, and other health science fields will consider articles on just about any topic that is remotely related to the aims of the journal.

Considering the primary audience for a manuscript is also important. For example, if the article's message is targeted to people working in a focused geographic area, a journal sponsored by a regional professional society that provides a copy of each issue to all members of the organization might be the best venue. Publishing in such a journal will ensure that the paper reaches those who will most benefit from it. On the other hand, if the study has conclusions that are relevant to an international audience, then a journal known to have a global readership might be more appropriate. However, the expansion of the Internet is making regional and international journals less distinct. Libraries and researchers nearly anywhere in the world are able to acquire copies of even relatively obscure publications.

One way to identify journals likely to consider a paper for publication is to examine the manuscript's reference list. The journals cited most often in the manuscript are likely to be suitable target journals. Abstract databases and library holdings may also provide a sense of which journals are likely to be interested.

■ 34.3 Impact Factors

The target journal should not be selected primarily because of its impact factor, ranking, or reputation, even though these are all factors to consider. The *impact factor* is based on the number of times a typical article in a journal is cited in its first year or two after publication. A few of the most prominent journals (like *Science, Nature, JAMA, The Lancet,* and the *New England Journal of Medicine*) have an impact factor of 10 or greater, but most journals in the health sciences have an impact factor closer to 1 or 2. Specialty journals may have an impact factor less than 1, but they can still be important within the specialty area. Impact factors are often listed on journal websites, and resources such as the Web of Knowledge (an electronic resource often available through university libraries) compile ratings for many journals.

■ 34.4 Journal Characteristics

After identifying potential journals, look at the journal requirements. For a review article, make sure that the target journal will accept reviews. Some journals specifically solicit short reports, which may allow authors a maximum of 1000 or 1500 words, one table or figure, and a limited number of references. These condensed manuscripts are an appealing option for a case report, a small case series, or an update to a previously published article. Alternatively, a comprehensive report of a large study that will exceed the usual 3000- or 3500-word limit or the standard limit of four tables and/or figures will require a journal that has more flexible word limits.

Some journals provide information about their turnaround time (the average time from submission to first decision) and/or their acceptance rates. Many big-name journals with low acceptance rates have a turnaround time of only a few days or weeks because they send very few manuscripts out for external review. Specialty journals with higher acceptance rates may have a turnaround time of several months because three or more external referees review nearly every manuscript.

Another consideration is the method of submission. Most journals have moved to online submission systems. These allow authors to upload manuscripts to a website and track the progress of their articles through the review process. Some journals ask authors to e-mail a copy of the paper to the editor, and some still require several copies of the paper to be sent by postal mail. Authors often prefer online systems because of the ability to monitor the status of their manuscripts, but this is not a priority for some researchers.

■ 34.5 Publication Costs

Although many journals are able to cover costs through subscriptions, advertising, and/or the support of a professional society, an increasing number of them are resorting to a variety of mechanisms that compel authors to cover some of the costs of publishing.

- A few journals require authors to pay a small *submission fee* and will not review an article until this payment is received.
- Some charge a small or large publication fee. The fee may be per article, usually called a *processing fee* or *processing charge*. Or the fee can be per article page, usually called a *page fee* or *page charge*. The number of pages is determined by the final ready-to-be-published article, not by the number of pages in the submitted manuscript.
- Some journals that are run by professional societies require the corresponding author of an accepted paper to become a member of the sponsoring society. In this situation, publication requires payment of a membership fee.
- Some journals require an *open access fee*, which allows the journal to make the article available online immediately upon publication with no restrictions.
- Some journals give authors the choice of whether they want to pay for open access. Researchers sponsored by funding agencies that require articles written with their support to be publicly available may thus pay for open access. Authors without funding may publish at no cost.

A few journals that charge fees may allow authors to request waivers of some fees if the authors are from low-income countries and/or if the project was not supported by a contract or grant. These requests usually must be made before the paper is reviewed. Publication fees are usually disclosed in a journal's author guidelines or somewhere else on the journal's website. Look for this information when considering publishing options.

■ 34.6 Online Journals

Some journals publish only print versions of their articles. However, the vast majority of print publications also offer online access to subscribers (usually libraries), even for articles that are not publicly available through an open access option. Articles published in these journals are assigned to an issue and given page numbers, but they are also available to subscribers as electronic files.

Some recently founded journals are available only online. Although many of these journals are likely to remain available online for many years to come, some researchers are wary about publishing in new, unproven journals that do not leave a paper trail. A subset of these new online open access journals have a reputation for not having rigorous review standards and being a sort of pay-to-publish scheme. In contrast, some open access online journals have quickly become well-respected journals that are regarded as having strong peer-review systems.

Before submitting to an online-only journal, be sure that the journal is legitimate and is indexed in relevant databases. For example, being indexed in a competitive database like MEDLINE, which examines the quality and editorial rigor of all candidate journals prior to accepting them for inclusion in the database, is validation of the journal's legitimacy.

The Submission, Review, and Publication Process

Manuscripts submitted to peer-reviewed journals are evaluated by editors and external reviewers, who provide feedback about how to improve a manuscript and make a decision about whether it is ready to be published.

■ 35.1 From Paper to Publication

Many brilliant and artfully written articles are published every year. And, every year, a lot of not-so-brilliant articles are published. A manuscript has a high likelihood of eventually being published if it is written in decent English (or written well in some other language), if the methods were reasonably rigorous and valid, and if the findings have a clear application or message.

Publication is a priority for many health researchers because, from the perspective of the broader scientific community, a project that has not been published is a project that never happened. Submitting to a journal as soon as a revised and polished manuscript has been crafted is critical. Procrastination can render the study useless because data in the health sciences quickly become obsolete and no longer publishable. (See Chapter 31 for writing strategies.) Submission is not the end of the writing process. Additional revisions will likely be required, even if the first journal to which a manuscript is submitted accepts the paper. This is another incentive to submit as soon as is reasonably possible: revising a manuscript is never easier than when the project is fresh in mind.

■ 35.2 Journal Selection

Once all coauthors are satisfied that the manuscript is ready to be submitted for peer review, *one* journal must be selected as the first journal for submission. Chapter 34 has suggestions for selecting an appropriate journal. A preliminary target journal may have been selected early in the research or writing process to serve as a guide. However, once a manuscript is completed, a variety of journals should again be considered. Only one can be selected as the first place to submit the completed manuscript.

Submitting to two or more journals at the same time is not permitted in the health sciences. Although editors of some popular magazines may compete for manuscripts from paid freelance authors, nearly all of the labor in the professional health journal system is voluntary. Editors may receive little or no compensation for their time, and reviewers and authors are unpaid volunteers. It would be a major strain on the editorial and review system if every manuscript was sent to several journals at the same time. Thus, most journals require a statement with each submitted manuscript affirming that the manuscript is under consideration only by that one journal. This rule should be assumed to be true for all journals. Once a manuscript has been submitted to a journal, it cannot be submitted elsewhere until either the authors are notified that it has been rejected or the authors formally withdraw it from consideration. The website of the Committee on Publication Ethics, whose membership includes the editors of several thousand biomedical journals, provides additional information about appropriate conduct for authors and the repercussions for those who violate standard protocols.

■ 35.3 Manuscript Formatting

Each journal provides *author guidelines* that state how manuscripts should be formatted. The guidelines must be carefully followed. See FIGURE 35-1 for examples of formatting preferences, which vary by journal.

Special attention should be paid to tables, figures, and other images when formatting the manuscript. The tables in the manuscript do not need to match the typographic style of the journal. Most journals will reformat the tables of all accepted manuscripts into their house styles when they convert the text into the single-spaced, small font, multicolumn format that is popular in health science journals.

However, graphs, maps, and other illustrations are rarely reworked by a journal's graphic designer prior to publication. So all figures should be polished prior to submission. Journals may require image files in a specific electronic format, which may or may not be a standard file type. Most journals charge a fee for printing color images but not for grayscale images. So use color only when it is absolutely necessary. (Alternatively, some journals charge for color in the print version but allow the online

Content	Should only the title be listed on the title page? Or should authors, word counts, key words, running headers (abbreviated versions of the title), or other information also be listed?
Author information	Should identifying information be blacked out in the manuscript (possibly including the citation information for references to previous works by the research team)? Or should author names be listed? Should authors' degrees, job titles, institutional affiliations, and/or contact information be listed?
Abstract/summary	Should the abstract be structured (showing subheadings for each section, such as "objective . . . methods . . . results . . . conclusion") or unstructured? If a structured abstract is expected, are there preferred subheadings? What is the word limit for the abstract? Should the abstract appear on its own page? Is an additional one-sentence summary or précis required? Are additional separate statements required, such as "what this paper will contribute to the literature"?
Keywords	How many keywords (search terms that will be linked to the article) should be provided? Must these be MeSH (medical subject heading) terms? Should these be listed somewhere in the manuscript?
Sections	Is there a preference for how sections within the document are labeled and formatted?
Acknowledgments/endmatter	Should acknowledgments of funding sources or personal assistance be included at the end of the manuscript? Is any additional endmatter to be included, such as information about the role of each coauthor, details about ethics committee review, declarations of potential conflicts of interest, or other disclosures?
In-text citation style	How should in-text references to works listed in the reference section be shown: as superscript numbers, as numbers within brackets, by the last name of the first author and the publication year in brackets or parentheses, by the names of several authors along with the publication year in brackets or parentheses, or by some other method? (Chapter 30 shows examples of these methods.)
Reference list order	Should the entries in the reference list be in alphabetical order (by the first author's last name) or in order of first appearance in the manuscript?

FIGURE 35-1 Manuscript Formatting Requirements Addressed by Journals' Author Guidelines

Reference style	What formatting does the journal require for the reference list? For example, how many authors should be listed for articles with more than 6 coauthors? Should the full journal title be listed or an abbreviation for the title? Should the issue and volume be listed, or just the volume? Should any of the parts of the reference be in bold or italics?
Page formatting	What margins and line spacing should be used? Do the lines on each page need to be numbered?
Page numbering	Should page numbers be shown at the bottom center of each page, the top right of each page, or elsewhere?
Fonts and font sizes	What fonts and font sizes should be used?
Word limits/page limits	What is the word limit or page limit? Does the word limit include only the main text of the article, or does it also include the abstract, references, and tables?
Tables and figures	Is the number of tables and/or figures limited? Should tables and figures appear in the manuscript following the paragraph in which they are first mentioned, or should they all be placed at the end of the manuscript file after the references? Should each table and figure be saved as a separate file, or should tables be left placed at the end of the manuscript file but figures saved as separate files?

FIGURE 35-1 (continued)

version of the manuscript to use color at no cost. In this situation, authors may submit a color version of the image but must make sure that the grayscale version has appropriate tones and adequate contrast.) Also, since an image may be resized prior to publication, check that each image can be enlarged or reduced without distortion.

■ 35.4 Cover Letter

Even though most submissions are made via computer instead of by postal delivery, most online submission systems still expect a cover letter to be uploaded. FIGURE 35-2 summarizes the content of a cover letter. The letter should summarize the manuscript and seek to convince the editor that the work is important, valid, original, and a good fit with the aims of the journal. Once submitted, the editorial staff's decision about whether to consider the article for publication may be made solely on the basis of the abstract and/or cover letter. So both of these items must be compelling.

Salutation	Address the letter to the editor(s) either generically ("Dear editor") or by name.
Basic information	Provide the title of the manuscript and, if the journal publishes different categories of articles, the type of article (such as original research, review, commentary, or short report).
Summary	Provide a short summary of the study design and key findings.
Importance	Make the case for why the manuscript is important, significant, and original.
Fit	Make the case for why the manuscript is a good fit for the journal.
Required declarations	Some journals require the cover letter to affirm that the manuscript is not under review elsewhere and has not been previously published, that all listed coauthors meet authorship criteria including the approval of submitting the manuscript to the journal, and/or that no conflicts of interest need to be disclosed to the editors. Some journals may additionally require information about the specific contributions of each coauthor and/or the funders of the research project.
Thanks	Thank the editors for considering the manuscript for possible review and publication.
Names/signatures	Some journals require the signatures of all authors to appear on the cover letter. A signed letter can be scanned into a computer and uploaded on the journal's submission website, or it can be faxed to the journal office.

FIGURE 35-2 **Sample Cover Letter Content**

■ 35.5 Online Submission

Once the manuscript files have been prepared and all the required supplemental information and materials have been compiled, the manuscript is ready to be submitted. The authors may need to send paper copies by postal mail, sometimes along with a computer disk containing the files. Alternatively, a journal might rejuice authors to e-mail the manuscript and cover letter to the journal. Most journals, however, require online submission.

Creating an account with a journal's submission website usually takes only a few minutes. Only the *corresponding author*—the coauthor who will communicate with the journal and answer questions from readers after the paper is published—needs to register. The corresponding author may be the first author, the senior coauthor, or the coauthor with the most stable e-mail address and affiliation. In addition to facilitating submission of the manuscript, the online account enables the corresponding author to track the manuscript's progress through the review process. Most online systems will indicate when the editorial office is considering an article, when the article is undergoing external review, and when a decision is pending. Online submission usually takes about half an hour, although it may be faster or slower depending on the amount of information requested and the number of steps in uploading.

Most submission websites start by asking for basic information about the article, such as the title, abstract, and keywords. The keywords may be able to be typed or pasted in, or they might be selected from a list provided by the journal. Some journals will also ask for:

- The type of article (such as original research, review article, or letter)
- The word count
- The number of tables
- The number of figures
- Statements about ethics approval, funding, possible conflicts of interest, and author contributions
- Confirmation that the article is being submitted to only one journal

A second step asks for information about all contributing authors. The corresponding author should check ahead of time with coauthors about the preferred forms of their names. Most authors in the health sciences choose to use a middle initial when publishing, since PubMed and several other abstract databases list authors by their last names and first and middle initials. Some journals also request a job title, affiliation, and contact information for all authors.

There may be additional steps. For example, the journal may request the names and contact information for three or more potential reviewers and/or a list of people who should not be reviewers because of a known conflict of interest. Some journals require a list of potential reviewers before a submission will be processed; some make this information optional.

The final step is uploading the manuscript files.

- Some journals require the title page to be uploaded separately from the rest of the manuscript, especially if they use double-blind review, in which reviewers are not told the names of authors and authors are not told the names of reviewers. (Some use single-blind review; reviewers are provided with the authors' names but authors are not provided with reviewers' names. Others use an open review process.)
- Many journals require each table and figure to appear in a separate file. The file types acceptable for figures vary among journals.
- The journal may request additional files, such as a publishing agreement signed by all authors or a checklist showing compliance with required contents and/or formats.

All of the manuscript files are typically combined into one pdf file during the submission process. The corresponding author should carefully review this file for completeness, page numbering, and the legibility of tables and figures prior to finalizing the submission. The author may also have an opportunity to review an html version of the uploaded paper and/or check the references for accuracy. (Some systems automatically link manuscript references to abstract databases so that reviewers can easily access the abstracts of the cited articles. Incorrect references may be flagged as having errors.) Once the manuscript and supporting files are confirmed to be correct, the submission is complete.

■ 35.6 Initial Review

Once a manuscript is submitted, the journal's editorial staff does a preliminary review and decides whether to send the manuscript to external peer reviewers or to reject it without review (FIGURE 35-3). Although the organizational structures of journals vary, typically the editor-in-chief who oversees the journal assigns new submissions to assistant editors for initial review. For manuscripts deemed worthy of review, the assistant editors identify *ad hoc* reviewers. These are reviewers who are not on the journal's editorial board who are asked to serve as peer reviewers because of their expertise on the paper's topic or methods. Some journals send nearly all manuscripts out to reviewers; others select only a small fraction of them for peer review.

Rejection without review (sometimes called a *desk rejection*) is often not a commentary on the quality of the manuscript. It is rather a decision based on the perceived fit of the paper with the journal's current interests. If an article is rejected without review, the authors should identify a different journal that might be a better fit, make

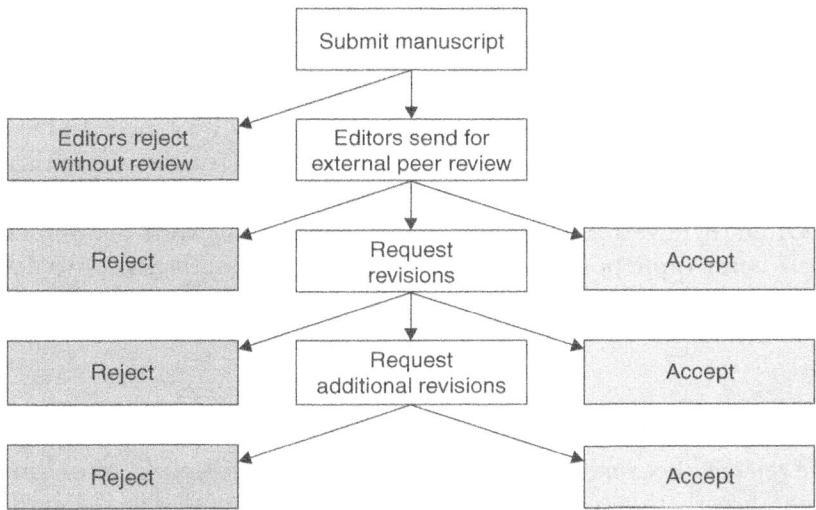

FIGURE 35-3 The Journal Review Process

any edits deemed necessary, reformat the manuscript for the new journal, and submit there.

One of the advantages of the initial review process is that it allows authors to quickly submit their work to a more suitable journal. Authors are often notified of a decision to reject without review within two weeks of submission, although in some situations notification may take three months or longer. When an article is selected for external review, notification usually takes at least two or three months, if not longer. Authors should usually not contact editorial offices to inquire about the status of their manuscript until at least four months after submission. Even then, a request for an update should be made only if the status of the paper has not recently been updated in the online submission management system.

■ 35.7 External Review Results

Decision letters sent after peer review are almost always accompanied by comments provided by one to four reviewers. Reviewers usually provide two sets of comments to the journal.

- The first set of comments is on the quality of the manuscript. These observations are intended to be shared with the authors and often include specific points that the authors should address to strengthen their manuscript.
- The second set of comments is intended only for the editor. Reviewers may be asked to rate the manuscript's novelty, importance, and fit with the journal in addition to the quality of the work.

An external peer review can lead to three possible results: rejection, an opportunity to revise and resubmit, or acceptance (Figure 35-3). An article determined to be methodologically sound and well written may receive low scores in the areas of interest or relevance to the journal. So it is possible for a manuscript to be rejected even if all the comments shared with authors are very positive. Alternatively, an article deemed to be somewhat lacking in writing quality may receive high scores for the originality of the topic and the apparent significance of the work, and may yield an invitation to revise and resubmit. Often reviews are mixed, with one or more reviewers being very critical and one or more being quite positive. Mixed reviews may lead the editor to decide either to reject the article or to offer the opportunity to revise and resubmit.

■ 35.8 Rejection

Some manuscripts are rejected because they are poorly written, incomplete, or of limited interest to those not directly involved in the project. However, many rejected manuscripts are well written, thorough, and interesting to a wide audience. Many journals have low acceptance rates and routinely reject high-quality papers. An appeal to the editor to reconsider a rejected manuscript will almost never result in a different outcome. So authors should simply put their energy into revising the manuscript for submission to another journal.

Rejection does not mean that the article has been rejected by all journals and will never be published anywhere. It simply means that one journal has decided that the paper is not suitable for its audience. Many authors find it helpful to take a few days to be disappointed about the rejection, to vent about some of the reviewer comments, and to complain about editorial decision making. But one rejection—or even several of them—does not mean that a paper will never be published. Each set of reviewer comments can strengthen a paper. Most papers are not fatally flawed, that is, so badly designed and conducted that they cannot be rescued. Most papers can be made suitable for publication somewhere, although gaining acceptance may require several weeks or several months of additional work. As long as researchers are willing to learn from each set of reviewer comments, the manuscript will continue to become stronger with each submission.

Begin work on revisions as soon as possible after receipt of a rejection letter. As time elapses after the completion of data collection and analysis, remembering the original aims, methods, and results becomes increasingly difficult. All reviewer comments should be read and carefully considered, with appropriate edits made. (The next section describes how to interpret reviewer comments.) Never submit to a second journal without taking advantage of the input provided by the first set of reviewers. For one thing, their feedback will improve the paper. For another, the manuscript may be sent to the same reviewers, who will not be happy if their evaluations were ignored. The revising process may require relatively little time, or it may demand significant reworking of entire sections of the manuscript. The background and discussion sections may need to be expanded to include more emphasis on the importance of the new paper and more citations of the relevant literature. The methods section may need to provide more details about the techniques used. The results section may need to show additional statistical output.

Once the manuscript has been edited to the satisfaction of all coauthors, a new target journal should be selected. The writing style and formatting of the paper may need to be updated to reflect the style of the new target journal prior to submission.

■ 35.9 Revision and Resubmission

When authors are invited to *revise and resubmit (R&R)* their manuscript to the same journal, they need to edit the manuscript and prepare a response to each reviewer comment. Authors may be given a deadline for resubmission. If they miss the deadline, the revised manuscript may be treated as a new submission and be sent out to new reviewers, which may significantly decrease the likelihood of acceptance. Some, but not all, journals make a distinction between a minor revision and a major revision. A *minor revision* may be reviewed only by the assistant editor after resubmission, whereas a *major revision* may be sent back to the original reviewers for a second look. A journal may allow only a very short time, perhaps three or four weeks, for a minor revision to be returned. A major revision may be given a deadline of three months or longer.

If the original reviewers are asked to re-review the manuscript, they will be provided with a copy of the authors' responses to their comments. Accordingly, every response needs to be carefully constructed and respectful. Examples of responses to comments are shown in FIGURE 35-4. Some reviewer suggestions—often marked as "minor"—will be easy to respond to, such as correcting typos, reformatting tables, or adding a few more citations. Others—often marked as "major"—may require more thought and time. Responding to comments that are complimentary or to points that the authors agree strengthen their papers is fairly easy.

Responding to critical comments is much more difficult. Authors who disagree with the suggestion of a reviewer are not obligated to change their paper to suit the reviewer, but they do need to write a thoughtful and conciliatory explanation of their point of view.

- Sometimes reviewer comments are hard to decipher or vague, such as "The entire manuscript is lacking focus and clarity." An appropriate response is to refer to exactly where and how the paper has been improved.
- Sometimes a reviewer's comments exhibit a lack of comprehension. Although it is tempting (and sometimes accurate) to assume that the reviewer was reading carelessly, the authors should consider how that part of the manuscript might be revised to promote clarity.
- Sometimes two reviewers offer conflicting advice. The responses to both of the comments should summarize both comments and explain how a decision was reached.

The response to reviewer comments should be prepared as a separate file from the manuscript. Additionally, some journals require a version of the manuscript that highlights or tracks the changes made in the document between the first submission and the resubmission. Once the revision is complete, a new cover letter, a revised manuscript, and the responses to reviewer comments can be uploaded to the journal submission website. The cover letter should thank the editors for the opportunity to revise and resubmit, thank the reviewers for their comments and state that their advice has improved the paper, and affirm that each reviewer comment has been reviewed and responded to.

The time needed for second review varies widely among journals, ranging from a few weeks to several months, depending on how many parties are involved in the re-review.

Sample Comment	Sample Response(s)
The specific aims of this paper should be clearly stated early in the manuscript.	We have edited the final paragraph of the introduction section to make it clear that the three specific aims of the paper are (1) to . . . , (2) to . . . , and (3) to . . . .
The paragraph on . . . is unclear.	We have rewritten this paragraph to improve clarity and to emphasize . . . .
Did your survey include a question about . . . ?	The data set we analyzed did not include a variable for . . . . However, even without that information, our analysis shows that . . . .
	This would have been a helpful question to ask, but, unfortunately, it was not included in our questionnaire.
	We did not ask this question in the baseline survey presented in this paper, but we do plan to ask a question about . . . in our follow-up study next year. We agree that this will be an interesting question to explore.
	We did ask this question and found . . . . We have added this finding to the results section.
	We did ask this question and found . . . .
The sample size seems too low to have adequate power for this study design.	We used . . . software before initiating our study to estimate our required sample size. With expected inputs of . . . and power of 80%, a sample size of . . . was estimated to be required. In total we recruited . . . participants. Based on the results of our study, and our estimates of power during data analysis, which showed . . . , our sample size is estimated to have sufficient power to yield significant results.
Table 3 seems incomplete. It should also report the results of the . . . test for each row.	We have done the additional analysis requested and have added a new column to Table 3 that shows the results of the . . . test. What we found was . . . , which is consistent with the results of our other statistical tests.
You used the . . . test to analyze . . . , but a . . . test would be more appropriate.	The . . . test that we used is the appropriate test because . . . . The alternate . . . test is not appropriate because . . . .
In the discussion section, the authors claim . . . , but is it possible that . . . is happening instead?	Our assertion that . . . is happening is based on . . . . This interpretation is supported by several recent publications, including . . . . We have expanded our rationale for this conclusion in the discussion section and added additional references to previous literature.
	The reviewer raises a very interesting point. We agree that both of these interpretations are possible, and now discuss both perspectives in the discussion section.

FIGURE 35-4 Sample Responses to Reviewer Comments

Sample Comment	Sample Response(s)
The conclusion about . . . is not supported by the data.	We have removed this claim. Our primary conclusion, which is fully supported by our results, is . . . .
You should include a discussion of	Thank you for raising this interesting point. We have added commentary on . . . to the discussion section.
	We agree that this is an interesting topic, but since . . . is only tangentially related to our specific aims, we do not have space to discuss it in this paper.
You need to add a paragraph on the limitations of the study.	We have added a paragraph on limitations to the discussion section.
Several recent publications have addressed the themes of your work and should be cited, including . . . , . . . , and	Thank you for bringing these articles to our attention. Both of the articles by . . . and . . . were helpful in supporting our findings and are now included as references.
I am not convinced that the study is important enough for publication in an international journal. It may be a better fit for a regional journal.	We have added an additional paragraph to the introduction that highlights what is new and significant about our findings. We have also added an additional paragraph to the discussion section that discusses the implications of our findings for other settings. We believe that our paper is important because . . . .
There are typos in lines . . . and . . . of page	Thank you for catching these typos. We have corrected both of them.

FIGURE 35-4 (continued)

35.10 After Acceptance

Papers are rarely accepted for publication as is, especially for a first submission. Acceptances are often *provisional acceptances* with final acceptance pending until a few minor adjustments to the manuscript are submitted. If a provisional acceptance is offered, journals will often ask that the required updates be made within a short period of time, sometimes in as little as one week. After the journal receives the corrected manuscript, a final acceptance letter will be sent to the corresponding author, usually by e-mail.

Once a paper is formally accepted, it is usually sent to a copyeditor, who checks the paper carefully for grammar, spelling, and adherence to the journal's style. (Some journals have a style manual for copyeditors that specifies the preferred phrases, terms, abbreviations, and spellings for articles published in that journal.) The paper is then sent to a layout specialist who formats the document to look like all the other articles published in the journal. The *page proofs* (or *galley proofs*) are then sent to the corresponding author for review, usually as a pdf file. Authors are usually given only one to three days to meticulously check the document, respond to any queries from the editor, and make any other editing requests. This is not the time to make any substantive changes; suggested corrections are limited to new problems, like formatting errors and copyedits that have changed the meaning of the text. However, read every line carefully, examine every figure for clarity and crispness, and check details like the spelling of authors' names, the contact information provided for the corresponding author, and the order of references. This is the last opportunity to catch errors.

After the authors return the page proofs, the time to publication of the article depends on the journal. Some journals will post a pdf file of the corrected page proofs on their websites as an *advance access* article or *preprint*. Others will not post the article online until it has been assigned to an issue and published in print form. An article may be published in an issue mere weeks after acceptance or many months after the page proofs are approved. Soon after the article is published, the abstract will be added to the databases that index the journal. The published article may be cited for the first time in another article about a year or so after publication. At this point, the research cycle is complete!

Why Publish?

Researchers take the time and effort to see a research project all the way to publication for many reasons.

■ 36.1 Scientific Dialogue

The peer-reviewed publication system (and, to a lesser extent, the professional conference network) is the primary way scientists communicate. Submitting a manuscript to
a journal for review is the first step in a series of conversations about the research project. The first back-and-forth conversation occurs with editors and reviewers. After the
article is published, the conversation continues as other researchers read, discuss, cite,
and apply the work. So, if the results of a research study are not published, for all
practical purposes it is as if the research was never done. The findings do not become
part of the conversation among scientists because there is no formal record of the project. Although the researcher may have learned from the project even if it is never formally written up, an unfinished report does not further scientific knowledge or improve
practice.

■ 36.2 Critical Feedback

The peer-review process is an important step toward producing a high-quality paper. Reviewers are usually quite adept at identifying weaknesses in an article and asking authors to carefully think through the problem areas and to respond to them. Responding to suggestions from editors and reviewers requires an author to:

- Understand and appreciate different perspectives
- Balance conflicting sets of advice about what would strengthen a paper
- Deal with the frustration of needing to rethink and rewrite whole portions of a paper to make the intended meaning clear (since unclear writing is usually at least partly to blame for reviewers who completely misread a part of a manuscript)
- Recover from a harsh review and move forward

Subjecting a manuscript to criticism and possible rejection can be intimidating and unpleasant, but the peer-review process produces stronger manuscripts and better scientists.

■ 36.3 Respect for Participants and Collaborators

If participants donate their time to a project, then the researcher has an ethical obligation to make sure that their time was not wasted. One way to fulfill this responsibility and to show respect for their contributions is to share the results of the study widely so that others learn from it.

If a project finds a significant association between an exposure and an outcome, that finding should become part of the scientific literature. If a project finds no association between an exposure and an outcome, the results may be even more important to publish so that other scientists do not waste their time and resources coming to the same conclusion. (Publishing a study with null results is often more challenging than publishing a study that finds an unexpected or strong association. However, a finding of no association is just as important as a finding of a statistically significant association as long as the study used valid methods.)

Seeing a project through to completion also shows respect for collaborators and mentors. Being a coauthor on an article or listed in the acknowledgments section is a reward or gesture of appreciation for everyone who assisted with the research process.

■ 36.4 A Step Toward Future Research

The research process does not necessarily end with a report. The research process is a cycle, in which data analysis and reporting naturally feed back into the formation of new study questions (FIGURE 36-1) and the establishment of a personal research trajectory. Publishing marks an important step in this cycle.

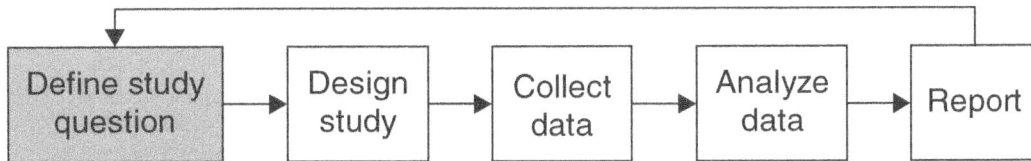

FIGURE 36-1 Each Research Project Raises New Questions to Be Explored in Future Projects

Publishing on the exact same topic twice is inappropriate. Redundant or duplicate publication is a violation of professional standards, and may result in the retraction of the articles. However, some aspects of the data set that were not covered in the first publication might be worth exploring. The newly published researcher should consider the related research projects that might be worth pursuing. The report probably identified a number of gaps in the literature that could be investigated. Furthermore, by contributing to the research literature, a published paper allows other health scientists to continue the research process by examining new study questions raised by the published report.

■ 36.5 Personal Benefits

Publishing enhances the authors' résumés/CVs. It indicates that a person is part of the scholarly community, can see a project through to completion, and has the ability to handle constructive criticism. A published article becomes a part of each author's permanent record; the paper will be indexed in abstract databases for decades and certainly for the length of each author's career. And, although authors of scholarly journal articles are not paid for their writing (and, in fact, are often happy when they do not have to pay publication fees), the payoff often comes in terms of improved job opportunities and promotions. Scientific publishing is unlikely to bring a person fame and fortune, but it does provide a tangible product after all the many hours that the author spent reading, planning, collecting data, running statistical analyses, and writing. A published paper is evidence of the author's professional expertise and commitment to improving health for individuals and communities.

Index

multivariate analysis, 211–220
  by study approach, 197–198
  confounding, 211–213
  dummy variables, 218–219
  interaction, 212–213
  linear regression, 214–217
  logistic regression, 217–218
  regression, 213–219
  survival analysis, 86, 219–220

N

narrative reviews, 37–38, 40
National Health and Nutrition
      Examination Survey
      (NHANES), 170
National Health Interview Survey
      (NHIS), 170
needs assessment, 54, 93
negative predictive value (NPV),
      88–89
−2 log likelihood test, 213
nested case–control studies, 111
newspapers, 15, 233
NLM reference style, 236
nominal variables, 128–129, 189
  comparative statistics, 207, 209
  descriptive statistics, 194–195
noninferiority trial, 80–81
nonmaleficence, 86, 151–153
nonparametric tests, 206
  comparative statistics, 207, 209
  correlation, 45–46
nonrandom-sampling bias, 107
non-response bias, 108
normal distribution, 192–193, 206
null hypothesis (H_0), 198–202, 207
null result, 175–176, 199, 278
number needed to harm (NNH), 86
number needed to treat (NNT),
      86–87
numeric variables, 127–128,
      188–190

O

observational studies, 78, 229
odds, 59–60
odds ratio (OR), 59–63, 203
one-sample median test, 207
one-sample t-test, 206–207
one-sided test, 201–202
one-way ANOVA, 207, 209
ongoing review, 166–167
online journals, 262

online submission, 261, 267–269
open access, 262
open-ended questions, 92, 127, 134
open review, 268
oral consent, 156
oral presentations, 250, 254–258
  concurrent sessions, 250
  question and answer time,
      257–258
  slide shows, 254–255
ordinal variables, 128–129, 189
  comparative statistics, 207, 209
  descriptive statistics, 194
ordinary least squares, 213
originality, 18–19
outcome variables, 213
outcomes
  for correlational studies, 44–45
  for cross-sectional surveys, 44–45
  for experimental studies, 79–81
  health outcomes, 11–12
outliers, 191, 195

P

page charge, 262
page fee, 262
page proofs, 274–275
paired data, 209–210
paired t-test, 209–210
paired-comparison questions, 128
panel studies, 69
parametric tests, 206
  comparative statistics, 207, 209
  correlation, 45–46
paraphrasing, 233–236
participant diaries, 92
participant observation, 91
participation rate, 140–142
  and estimated sample size, 121
  and incentives, 154
  and study population, 108
patient charts, 51, 171–172
Pearson correlation coefficient (r),
      45–46
peer review, 269–274, 278
person-place-time, 50–51, 57, 224
person-time, 71–72
phenomenology, 91
photographs, 227
physical fitness tests, 150
physiological function tests, 149
pie chart, 193–194
pilot test, 137

placebo, 81–83, 114
placebo effect, 81
plagiarism, 195, 233–236
plenary sessions, 250
pooled statistic in meta-analysis,
      176–177
Population Reference Bureau, 16
population research, 2–3
populations, 12
positive predictive value (PPV),
      88–89
postal surveys, 139–140
poster presentations, 250, 251–253
  poster content, 251
  poster layout, 252–253
  poster sessions, 250, 253
power ($1–\beta$), 121–122
précis, 245
predictor variables, 213
pregnant women, 114
preprints, 275
pretest, 137
prevalence, 54
prevalence rate ratio (PRR), 54
prevalence surveys (*See* cross-
      sectional studies)
primary investigator (PI), 100
primary studies, 21–22, 34–35
  ethical considerations, 151–168
  funding, 99
  interviews, 139–144
  proposals, 101–102
  protocols, 102–103
  questionnaire design, 125–135
  questionnaire validation, 136,
      137
  recruiting, 140–142
  research plan, 98
  research populations, 105–108
  sample size, 117–121
  self-administered surveys,
      139–144
  timelines, 100
PRISMA checklist, 229
prisoners, 114, 154
privacy, 157–158
processing charge, 262
processing fee, 262
program evaluation, 54, 93
project evaluation, 54, 93
proportionate mortality rate, 52
proportions, 207
proposal, 97, 101–102

simple randomization, 84
single-blind study, 83
skew, 192
skips
  in paper-based surveys, 134–135
  in computer-assisted surveys, 130, 135, 143
  in data entry programs, 183
snowballing, 174
socioeconomic position (SEP), 11
socioeconomic status (SES), 11
source population, 105–106
  and confidence intervals, 202–203
spatial analysis, 150, 220
Spearman rank order correlation (r, ρ), 45–46
specific aims, 22–23
specific hypotheses, 22–23
specific knowledge, 235
specific objectives, 22–23
specificity, 88–89
spread, 191–195
standard deviation, 192–193
  and coding for missing information, 183
  and comparative tests, 206–207
  and sample size, 119
  and z-score, 193
standard error, 215–218
standard of care, 81–82
statistical honesty, 195
statistical power $(1-\beta)$, 121–122
stepwise model, 213
stratified randomization, 84–85
stratified sampling, 107
STROBE checklist, 229
structured abstract, 223
study goals, 22–23
study population, 105–106, 108
submission fee, 262
submission of a manuscript, 261, 267–269
summary statistic in meta–analysis, 176–177
superiority trial, 79–80
surveillance, 69, 164

survival analysis, 86, 219–220
SWOT analysis, 93
systematic reviews, 37–38, 40, 173–178
  data extraction, 175–176
  eligibility criteria, 174–175
  research process, 38
  search strategy, 174
  topic selection, 39, 173–174
  writing checklist, 229
systematic sampling, 107

T
tables, 226–227
target journal, 259–262, 264
target population, 105–106
tau (τ), 46
telephone interviews, 139–141, 156
tertiary studies, 21–22, 34–35, 173–179
  research plan, 98
  systematic reviews, 37–38, 40, 173–176
  meta-analyses, 37–38, 40–41, 176–178
test of comprehension, 156
third variable effects, 211–213
time series, 69
timelines, 35–36, 100, 162
topic mapping, 9–10
transcription, 92
translation, 136–137, 159
treatment-assigned analysis, 86–88
treatment-received analysis, 86–88
TREND checklist, 229
t-test, 207–208, 209
2 × 2 table
  for cohort studies, 74–75
  for experimental studies, 87
  for matched case-control studies, 62–63
  for screening tests, 88–89
  for unmatched case-control studies, 59–60
  recoding for analysis, 204–205
two-sample t-test, 207–208
two-sided test, 201–202

type 1 error, 121–122
type 2 error, 121–122

U
UNDP, 16
UNICEF, 16
uniform distribution, 192
Uniform Requirements for Manuscripts Submitted to Biomedical Journals, 26–27
unimodal distribution, 192
univariate analysis, 187–195
unstructured abstract, 223

V
validation, 136
values, 4, 10
Vancouver reference style, 236
variability, 191, 214–218
variables, 127–129, 188–190
verbal consent, 156
voluntariness, 85, 153–154
vulnerable populations, 114, 159–160

W, X, Y, Z
waiver of consent, 158
Web of Knowledge, 261
Web of Science, 16
websites, 15, 232–233
weight, 148, 159
white space, 134, 252
Wilcoxon rank sum test, 207
Wilcoxon signed-rank test, 209
Wilcoxon-Mann-Whitney test, 207
word limits, 223, 241, 261
World Bank, 16
World Health Organization (WHO), 15, 16, 170
writer's block, 242–243
writing groups, 26, 241
writing strategies, 239–243
writing style, 233–234, 247–248
written consent, 156
z-score, 193

CPSIA information can be obtained at www.ICGtesting.com
Printed in the USA
LVOW03s0318150115

422902LV00025B/1046/P

9 781284 071603